AF567041

Research Projects in Dry Eye Syndrome

Developments in Ophthalmology

Vol. 45

Research Projects in Dry Eye Syndrome

Volume Editor

Horst Brewitt Hannover

54 figures, 1 in color, and 8 tables, 2010

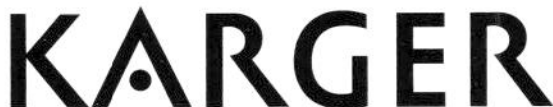

Basel · Freiburg · Paris · London · New York · Bangalore · Bangkok · Shanghai · Singapore · Tokyo · Sydney

Horst Brewitt
Ubbenstrasse 11
DE–30159 Hannover

This book was generously supported by

Alcon® and BAUSCH + LOMB

Library of Congress Cataloging-in-Publication Data

Research projects in dry eye syndrome / volume editor, Horst Brewitt.
p. ; cm. -- (Developments in ophthalmology, ISSN 0250-3751 ; v. 45)
Includes bibliographical references and index.
ISBN 978-3-8055-9418-9 (hard cover : alk. paper)
1. Dry eye syndromes. I. Brewitt, H. (Horst) II. Series: Developments in ophthalmology, v. 45. 0250-3751 ;
[DNLM: 1. Dry Eye Syndromes. W1 DE998NG v.45 2010 / WW 208 R432 2010]
RE216.D78R47 2010
617.7'1--dc22
2010007067

www.karger.com
Printed in Switzerland on acid-free and non-aging paper (ISO 9706) by Reinhardt Druck, Basel
ISSN 0250–3751
ISBN 978–3–8055–9418–9
e-ISBN 978–3–8055–9419–6

Contents

List of Contributors

Caroline A. Blackie, Dr.
Korb Associates
400 Commonwealth Ave.
Unit 2
Boston, MA 02215 (USA)
E-Mail cblackie@tearscience.com

Horst Brewitt, Prof. Dr.
Ubbenstrasse 11
DE–30159 Hannover (Germany)
E-Mail HorstBrewitt@T-Online.de

Meral Bulgen
Department of Ophthalmology
Ludwig Maximilian University
Mathildenstrasse 8
DE–80336 Munich (Germany)
E-Mail meral.bulgen@yahoo.de

Matthias Dunse
Department of Anatomy and Cell Biology
Martin Luther University Halle-Wittenberg
Grosse Steinstrasse 52
DE–06097 Halle/Saale (Germany)
E-Mail info@matthiasdunse.de

Markus Frentz
Department of Ophthalmology
RWTH Aachen University
Pauwelsstraße 30
DE–52074 Aachen (Germany)
E-Mail frentz@acto.de

Thomas A. Fuchsluger, Dr.
Department of Ophthalmology
University of Duisburg-Essen
Hufelandstrasse 55
DE–45122 Essen (Germany)
E-Mail thomas.fuchsluger@uk-essen.de

Fabian Garreis
Department of Anatomy and Cell Biology
Martin Luther University Halle-Wittenberg
Grosse Steinstrasse 52
DE–06097 Halle/Saale (Germany)
E-Mail fabian.garreis@medizin.uni-halle.de

Gerd Geerling, Prof. Dr.
Klinik für Augenheilkunde
Julius Maximilians Universität Würzburg
Josef-Schneider-Str. 11
DE–97080 Würzburg
E-Mail G.Geerling@augenklinik.uni-wuerzburg.de

U. Gehlsen, Dr.
Department of Ophthalmology
University Medical Center Schleswig-Holstein
Campus Lübeck, Ratzeburger Allee 160
DE–23538 Lübeck (Germany)
E-Mail gehlsen@anat.uni-luebeck.de

Jürgen Giebel, Prof. Dr.
Institute of Anatomy and Cell Biology
Ernst-Moritz-Arndt University
Friedrich-Loeffler-Str. 23c
DE–17487 Greifswald (Germany)
E-Mail giebel@uni-greifswald.de

Maria Gottschalt, Dr.
Department of Anatomy and Cell Biology
Martin Luther University Halle-Wittenberg
Grosse Steinstrasse 52
DE–06097 Halle/Saale (Germany)
E-Mail maria.gottschalt@web.de

Jutta Horwath-Winter, Dr.
Department of Ophthalmology
Medical University of Graz
Auenbruggerplatz 4
AT–8036 Graz (Austria)
E-Mail jutta.horwath@medunigraz.at

Gereon Hüttmann, Dr.
Biomedical Optics
University of Lübeck
Peter-Monnik-Weg 4
DE–23562 Lübeck (Germany)
E-Mail huettmann@bmo.uni-luebeck.de

Kristin Jäger, Dr.
Department of Anatomy and Cell Biology
Martin Luther University Halle-Wittenberg
Grosse Steinstrasse 52
DE–06097 Halle/Saale (Germany)
E-Mail kristin.jaeger@medizin.uni-halle.de

Clemens Jürgens, Dr.
Klinik für Augenheilkunde
Ernst-Moritz-Arndt-Universität Greifswald
Ferdinand-Sauerbruch-Strasse
DE–17475 Greifswald (Germany)
E-Mail juergens@uni-greifswald.de

Anselm Kampik, Prof. Dr.
Augenklinik der LMU
Klinikum der Universität München
Campus Innenstadt
Mathildenstrasse 8
DE–80336 Munich (Germany)
E-Mail akampik@med.uni-muenchen.de

Karsten Kasper
Department of Ophthalmology
Julius Maximilian University Würzburg
Josef-Schneider-Straße 11
DE–97080 Würzburg (Germany)
E-Mail k-augen@augenklinik.uni-wuerzburg.de

Sieglinde Kirchengast
Department of Ophthalmology
Medical University of Graz
Auenbruggerplatz 4
AT–8036 Graz (Austria)
E-Mail sieglinde.kirchengast@medunigraz.at

Erich Knop, Dr.
Research Laboratory of the Department of Ophthalmology CVK
Charité – Universitätsmedizin Berlin
Ziegelstrasse 5–9
DE–10117 Berlin (Germany)
E-Mail erich.knop@charite.de

Nadja Knop, Dr.
Department of Cell Biology in Anatomy
Hannover Medical School
Carl-Neuberg-Strasse 1
DE–30625 Hannover (Germany)
E-Mail knopnadja@aol.com

Donald R. Korb, Prof. Dr.
Korb Associates
400 Commonwealth Ave.
Unit 2
Boston, MA 02215 (USA)
E-Mail drkorb@aol.com

L. Liu, Dr.
Academic Unit of Ophthalmology
Institute of Biomedical Research
College of Medical and Dental Sciences
University of Birmingham
GB–B15 2TT Birmingham (UK)
E-Mail leiliudang@googlemail.com

Daniel Meller, Prof. Dr.
Department of Ophthalmology
University of Duisburg-Essen
Hufelandstrasse 55
DE–45122 Essen (Germany)
E-Mail daniel.meller@uk-essen.de

Elisabeth M. Messmer, Dr.
Department of Ophthalmology
Ludwig Maximilian University
Mathildenstrasse 8
DE–80336 Munich (Germany)
E-Mail emessmer@med.uni-muenchen.de

Mikk Pauklin, Dr.
Department of Ophthalmology
University of Duisburg-Essen
Hufelandstrasse 55
DE–45122 Essen (Germany)
E-Mail mikkpauklin@gmail.com

Friedrich P. Paulsen, Prof. Dr.
Department of Anatomy II
University of Erlangen-Nürnberg
Universitätsstraße 19
DE-91054 Erlangen
E-Mail friedrich.paulsen@anatomie2.med.uni-erlangen.de

Dieter Franz Rabensteiner, Dr.
Department of Ophthalmology
Medical University of Graz
Auenbruggerplatz 4
AT–8036 Graz (Austria)
E-Mail dieter.rabensteiner@medunigraz.at

Robert Rath, Dr.
Klinik für Augenheilkunde
Ernst-Moritz-Arndt-Universität Greifswald
Ferdinand-Sauerbruch-Strasse
DE–17475 Greifswald (Germany)
E-Mail rath.r@freenet.de

Otto Schmut, Prof. Dr.
Department of Ophthalmology
Medical University of Graz
Auenbruggerplatz 4
AT–8036 Graz (Austria)
E-Mail otto.schmut@medunigraz.at

Stefan Schrader, Dr.
Cells for Sight Transplantation and Research Programme
Department of Ocular Biology and Therapeutics
UCL Institute of Ophthalmology
11–43 Bath Street
GB–EC1V 9EL London (UK)
E-Mail mail@stefanschrader.de

Norbert F. Schrage, Prof. Dr.
Department of Ophthalmology
RWTH Aachen University
Pauwelsstraße 30
DE-52074 Aachen (Germany)
E-Mail schrage@acto.de

Ute Schulze
Department of Anatomy and Cell Biology
Martin Luther University
Grosse Steinstrasse 52
DE–06097 Halle/Saale (Germany)
E-Mail ute.schulze@medizin.uni-halle.de

Saadettin Sel, Dr.
Department of Ophthalmology
Martin Luther University
Grosse Steinstrasse 52
DE–06097 Halle/Saale (Germany)
E-Mail saadettin.sel@medizin.uni-halle.de

Felix Spöler, Dr.
Institute of Semiconductor Electronics
RWTH Aachen University
Sommerfeldstrasse 24
DE–52074 Aachen (Germany)
E-Mail spoeler@iht.rwth-aachen.de

Eva Spreitzhofer, Dr.
Department of Ophthalmology
Medical University of Graz
Auenbruggerplatz 4
AT–8036 Graz (Austria)
E-Mail eva_spreitzhofer@yahoo.de

Clark Springs, Dr.
Department of Ophthalmology
Indiana University
200 W. 103rd Street No. 2200
Indianapolis, IN 46290 (USA)
E-Mail csprings@iupui.edu

Klaus-Peter Steuhl, Prof. Dr.
Department of Ophthalmology
University of Duisburg-Essen
Hufelandstrasse 55
DE–45122 Essen (Germany)
E-Mail Klaus-Peter.Steuhl@uk-essen.de

Philipp Steven, Dr.
Department of Ophthalmology
University Medical Center Schleswig-Holstein
Campus Lübeck, Ratzeburger Allee 160
DE–23538 Lübeck (Germany)
E-Mail p.steven@uk-sh.de

Frank Tost, Prof. Dr.
Klinik und Poliklinik für Augenheilkunde
Ernst-Moritz-Arndt-Universität Greifswald
Ferdinand-Sauerbruch-Strasse
DE–17475 Greifswald (Germany)
E-Mail tost@uni-greifswald.de

Gabriele Trummer
Department of Ophthalmology
Medical University of Graz
Auenbruggerplatz 4
AT–8036 Graz (Austria)
E-Mail gabriele.trummer@medunigraz.at

Christine Wachswender
Department of Ophthalmology
Medical University of Graz
Auenbruggerplatz 4
AT–8036 Graz (Austria)
E-Mail christine.wachswender@medunigraz.at

Henrike Westekemper, Dr.
Department of Ophthalmology
University of Duisburg-Essen
Hufelandstrasse 55
DE–45122 Essen (Germany)
E-Mail henrike.westekemper@uk-essen.de

Torsten Witte, Prof. Dr.
Klinik für Immunologie und Rheumatologie
Medizinische Hochschule Hannover
Carl-Neuberg-Strasse 1
DE–30625 Hannover (Germany)
E-Mail witte.torsten@mh-hannover.de

Preface

Dedicated to Prof. Behrens-Baumann on His 65th Birthday

Dry eye is one of the most clinically established eye diseases worldwide. Over the last 40 years, our knowledge of this complex disease pattern has improved substantially. The official 2007 report of the International Dry Eye WorkShop is an encyclopedic review of this disease, which comprehensively summarizes our current knowledge of the pathogenesis, clinical signs, diagnostics and therapy. Nevertheless, it is essential to remain open to new research and continue to pose questions in this field.

Therefore, over the last few years in Germany, the Ressort Trockenes Auge (linked with the Professional Association of German Ophthalmologists – BVA) has regularly supported research projects on dry eye disease and other related diseases of the ocular surface.

Prof. Behrens-Baumann, director of the Universitäts-Augenklinik Magdeburg (University of Magdeburg Eye Clinic), is an active member of this independent scientific committee and has played a large role in its activities.

Theoretical and clinical research has formed a significant part of his career and of the clinic's activities. With this in mind, we have started to initiate and promote joint research projects with young scientists aimed at investigating the complex disease pattern of dry eye and other diseases of the ocular surface.

For this reason, I wish to dedicate this book to Prof. Behrens-Baumann on the occasion of his 65th birthday. Within these pages, well-respected German-speaking scientists working in university clinics have clearly and extensively presented their current research projects. The wide ranging themes vary from experimental basic research through to clinical practices for dry eyes. This excellent contribution makes it clear to the reader that we can look forward to exciting and stimulating research in the future.

I would like to thank all the authors for their willingness to participate in this project. In this way, you have shown your appreciation towards Prof. Behrens-Baumann.

On his 65th birthday, we wish Prof. Behrens-Baumann all the best and, above all, health and joie de vivre. May he be able to further develop his many musical and artistic interests in the future, as he has done during his professional life.

Acknowledgments

Special thanks goes to Alcon Pharma (Freiburg) and Bausch & Lomb – Dr. Mann Pharma (Berlin) for their financial support which helped make this book a reality.

The Dry Eye Research Award of the Ressort Trockenes Auge within the BVA is sponsored by Bausch & Lomb – Dr. Mann Pharma, who at this point I would like to thank for 10 years of generous financial support.

Last, but by no means least, I would like to thank Karger Publishers for the successful production of this 'birthday book'.

Horst Brewitt, Hannover
May 2010

Brewitt H (ed): Research Projects in Dry Eye Syndrome.
Dev Ophthalmol. Basel, Karger, 2010, vol 45, pp 1–11

Trefoil Factor Family Peptide 3 at the Ocular Surface. A Promising Therapeutic Candidate for Patients with Dry Eye Syndrome?

U. Schulze[a] · S. Sel[b] · F.P. Paulsen[a]

Departments of [a]Anatomy and Cell Biology and [b]Ophthalmology, Martin Luther University Halle-Wittenberg, Halle/Saale, Germany

Abstract

Dry eye syndrome is a widespread disease accompanied by discomfort and potential visual impairments. Basic causes are tear film instability, hyperosmolarity of the tear film, increased apoptosis as well as chronic inflammatory processes. During the last decades, our understanding of dry eye syndrome has considerably increased. However, the molecular mechanisms of the disease remain largely elusive. In this context, our group focuses on trefoil factor 3 (TFF3). Among other factors, TFF3 performs a broad variety of protective functions on surface epithelium. Its main function seems to be in enhancing wound healing by promoting a process called 'restitution'. Studies evaluating TFF3 properties and effects at the ocular surface using in vivo as well as in vitro models have revealed a pivotal role of TFF3 in corneal wound healing. Subsequent studies in osteoarthritic cartilage seem to draw a different picture of TFF3, which still needs further elucidation. This manuscript summarizes the findings concerning TFF3 in general and its role in the cornea as well as articular cartilage – two tissues which have some things in common. It also discusses the potential of TFF3 as a candidate therapeutic agent for the treatment of, for example, ocular surface disorders.

The ocular surface is constantly exposed to the external environment, and hence epithelial defects caused by injuries, infections as well as diseases may occur. Modern living has given rise to a massive increase in the incidence of vision-threatening dry eye disease; around 10–30% of the population living in industrialized countries suffer from dry eye syndrome [1]. According to the definition of the Dry Eye Workshop Study Group in 2007 [2], dry eye disease is 'a multifactorial disease of the tears and ocular surface that results in symptoms of discomfort, visual disturbances, and tear film instability with potential damage to the ocular surface. It is accompanied by increased osmolarity of the tear film and inflammation of the ocular surface.' Reduced production of tear fluid or changes in the tear film composition with impaired tear film stability results in diminished moistening of the ocular surface with tear fluid.

Consequently, this leads to several aftereffects, like inflammation, adaptive immune reaction (including T cell activation), apoptosis and bacterial colonization [2]. To cope with these challenges and ensure clear vision, a rapid wound healing process is necessary at the ocular surface.

Over the past 10 years, the trefoil factor family (TFF) and in particular one of its members, trefoil factor 3 (TFF3), has edged ever closer to the spotlight – particularly since TFF3 was found to promote healing processes in the organism, especially in the mucus layer lining the gastrointestinal tract. The ocular surface is also a mucosal surface. When considered together with the protective properties of TFF3, this gives rise to the hypothesis that TFF3 is a promising therapeutic agent for ocular surface defects and especially for dry eye syndrome [3].

TFF Peptides in General and TFF3 in Particular

The trefoil factor family consists of 3 family members: TFF1 (formerly pS2), TFF2 (formerly hSP) and TFF3 (formerly hP1.B/hITF). They are characterized by a trefoil domain of 38–41 amino acids which contains 6 conserved cysteine residues. These 6 amino acids form 3 disulfuric bonds in a Cys1-Cys5, Cys2-Cys4, Cys3-Cys6 configuration [4]. Thus, a very rigid so-called 'trefoil structure' is formed, which offers relative protection to these peptides from proteolytic degradation. Both TFF1 and TFF3 have one trefoil domain, but form dimers by a fourth intermolecular disulfuric bond. TFF2 on the other hand has a monomeric structure, but consists of two trefoil domains.

The TFF peptides are mucus associated, and show a tissue-specific expression pattern. Until now, they have been detected in the gastrointestinal tract [5], salivary glands [6], uterus and endocervix [7] as well as the mamma [8] and as a secretory component in human milk [9]. Furthermore, TFF peptides have been found in the respiratory tract [10], colocalized with oxytocin in hypothalamic cells [11], in Vater's ampulla [12], esophageal submucosal glands [13] as well as several other tissues [14].

At the ocular surface and the lacrimal apparatus, expression of TFF1 and TFF3 has been identified in goblet cells of the conjunctiva [15, 16] as well as in epithelial cells of the lacrimal sac and nasolacrimal sac [17]. Moreover, TFF peptides have been shown to play a role in dacryolith formation within the nasolacrimal passage. Interestingly, TFF2 is present in dacryoliths, while it is normally absent from the efferent tear duct system [18]. With regard to the ocular surface, TFF3 mRNA expression was present in healthy cornea, whereas at the protein level no TFF3 could be detected. However, under corneal pathological conditions – like Fuchs dystrophy, herpetic keratitis, keratoconus as well as pterygium – TFF3 protein was detectable [19]. Furthermore, it has been shown by in vivo studies that TFF3 protein is induced after corneal epithelial injuries in mice [20].

Although a lot of TFF3-binding proteins have been characterized, the receptor that mediates TFF3 signaling has not yet been identified [21]. It is assumed that the receptor is localized at the basolateral side of the cell membrane in epithelial cells, and is exposed only after defects in the mucus (fig. 1) [3, 5]. Recently, the low-affinity chemokine receptor CXCR4 has been identified as a receptor for TFF2 [22]. However, TFF3 should be considered as potential ligand for that receptor as well [23].

It is known that TFF peptides offer a broad variety of protective functions [14]. They directly interact with mucins and thereby influence the rheology of the mucus in general and tear fluid in particular [24–26]. Recent ex vivo studies with tear fluid from patients with dry eye syndrome seem to support this theory. In these experiments, a positive influence of recombinant human TFF3 peptide applied into the patient's tear fluid has been observed (unpublished data). Furthermore, TFF peptides participate in the packaging and secretion of mucins. The latter demonstrates the close correlation between mucins and TFF peptides, as well as the close cooperation of TFF peptides with other proteins in general [4]. Along with their contribution in the immune response [27, 28], they are also linked to tumor progression [29, 30].

TFF3 in particular shows anti-apoptotic characteristics [31–33], promotes human airway epithelial ciliated cell differentiation [34] and has motogenic properties [5]. Several groups have observed that TFF3 enhances the migration of epithelial cells into the surrounding areas [35–38]. Moreover, TFF3 plays a key role in the process of restitution. Once the surface integrity of the epithelial layer is impaired by a defect or an injury, cells of the surrounding unaffected tissue detach from the united cell structure and migrate into the affected area. This critical early phase of the migration ensures rapid re-epithelialization [39]. Studies with murine trefoil factor 3 knock-out mice ($Tff3^{-/-}$) have shown that TFF3 is essential for restitution, since these mice showed an impaired wound healing process [20, 40].

TFF3 at the Ocular Surface

At the ocular surface, Göke et al. [35] demonstrated the wound healing potential of recombinant TFF3 in vitro in primary rabbit corneal epithelial cells. Ensuing in vivo or combined in vivo-in vitro studies in two established corneal defect mouse models led to consistent and even more interesting results [20]. Corneal defects were induced by alkali burns (0.5 M NaOH) or by excimer laser ablation, resulting in severe localized impairment and removal of the corneal epithelium, whereas the corneal stroma and endothelium remained unaffected. To identify the endogenous expression pattern, murine Tff3 protein expression was then analyzed at different time points after the lesion. As in the healthy human cornea [19], Tff3 was absent in normal murine corneal tissue, but had already been induced in the corneal epithelium 1 h after injury. After the lesion, Tff3 expression levels in the cells close to the defect area gradually increased; even after wound closure, protein levels remained relatively high in the epithelial cells. Conversely, stromal and endothelial cells were Tff3-negative at all observed time points. Inducible expression results after injury support the protective

Fig. 1. TFF3 receptor hypothesis. The TFF3 receptor is assumed to be localized in the basolateral side of the cell membrane of epithelial cells within the mucus layer. It is exposed to its ligands only after defects. Modified from Paulsen [3].

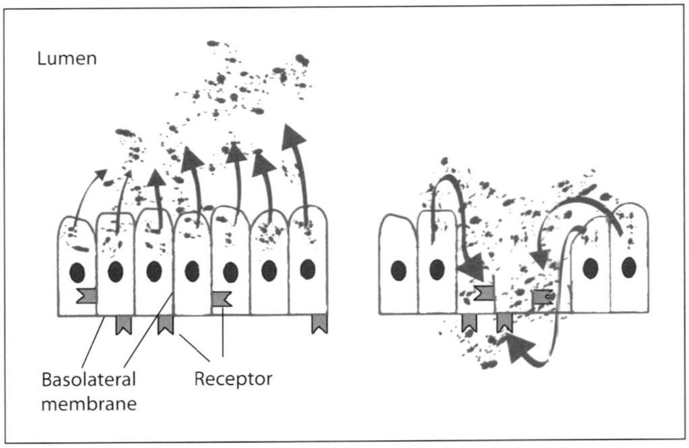

role of TFF3. This correlates with the findings that in Tff3$^{-/-}$ knockout mice corneal healing is prolonged after alkali burns as well as excimer-laser-induced injuries. Wild-type mice recover from these defects after approximately 10 h, whereas in knockout mice re-epithelialization was prolonged up to 462 h. Along with this difference in healing time, the hypothesis of Tff3 playing a pivotal role is also underlined by the finding that the recovered corneal epithelium was reduced in size and quality in 50% of the knockout mice. Only a monolayer of cells could be detected in these mice, and several areas showed detachment of the epithelium from the stroma as well as infiltration with immune cells, mainly lymphocytes. Furthermore, Tff3$^{-/-}$ mice lack Tff3 secreted into the tear film by conjunctival goblet cells (in addition to inducible corneal peptide), which would be provided to the apical corneal epithelium in wild-type mice.

In order to verify the in vivo results, experiments were also performed in a combined in vivo-in vitro model. First, the standardized alkali-induced corneal defects were allowed to partially heal in vivo for 6 h. Afterwards, mice were sacrificed, bulbi were enucleated, pinned down on dental wax and further cultured in a 24-well plate for an additional 124 h. The healing process was observed by measuring the remaining wounded area. Similar to in vivo results, a decelerated corneal recovery was observed in Tff3$^{-/-}$ mice bulbi in comparison to wild-type mice bulbi (fig. 2). The difference in recovery time was around 20 h, which is still a big difference since normal murine corneal recovery is a very rapid process.

To evaluate the biological effect of exogenously applied TFF3 upon in vivo corneal healing, ocular surface defects were induced by placing an alkali-soaked filter disk (2 mm) onto the cornea for 2 min or by excimer laser ablation following ophthalmic drop medications 3 times a day for a period of 3 days. These drops contained exogenous recombinant human TFF3 (rhTFF3) in different concentrations or bovine serum albumin (BSA) as a nonspecific protein control. Wound healing was analyzed at two

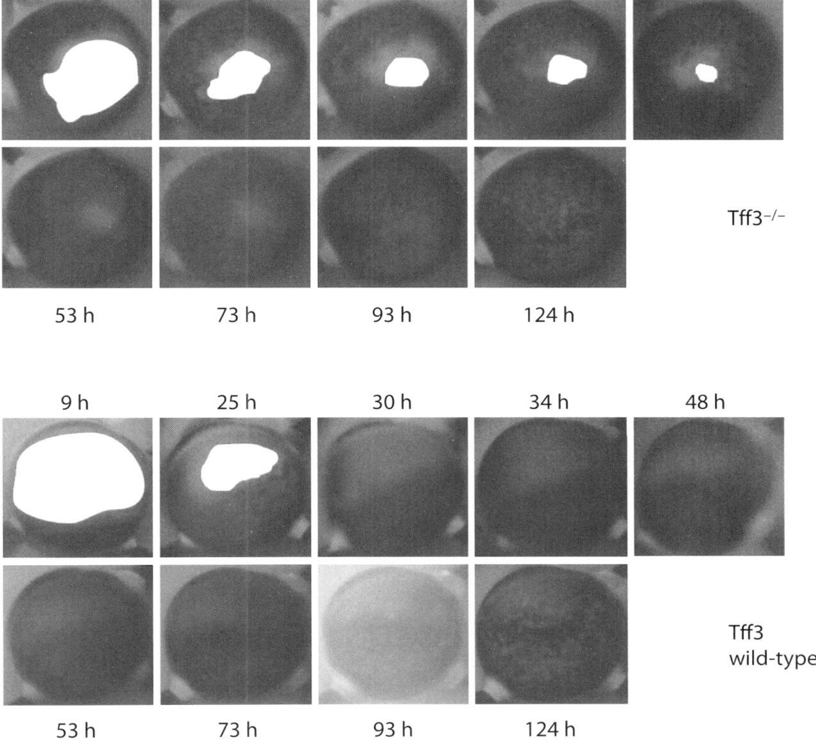

Fig. 2. Tff3$^{-/-}$ mice show decelerated corneal wound healing. Alkali-induced defects in Tff3$^{-/-}$ mice as well as in wild-type mice were allowed to partially heal in vivo for 6 h, followed by further in vitro cultivation for up to 124 h. Photographs were taken after 9, 25, 30, 34, 48, 53, 73, 93 and 124 h, and analysis of the wounded area was performed by measuring the remaining defect area using photo software. For better visualization, corneal defects are marked in white. Wound closure was completed after 30 h in wild-type mice, whereas in Tff3$^{-/-}$ knockout mice healing was finished after around 53 h (taking around 20 h longer). Modified from Paulsen et al. [20].

different time points using a grading system. The treated eyes were grouped according to the remaining impairments in the wounded area, such as defect extent and intensity, inflammatory environment observed by conjunctival hyperemia, and light reflection as a sign for identifying smoothness of the ocular surface. Three categories were considered: healed, moderately healed, and defect still present. It was obvious that rhTFF3 promoted the wound healing process in a dose-dependent manner (fig. 3). The highest concentrations (5 mg/ml rhTFF3 for alkali-induced defects and 10 mg/ml rhTFF3 for excimer laser-induced defects) accelerated the recovery process best, followed by a lower dose of rhTFF3 application, compared to BSA controls.

In order to verify these data, the experiments were repeated in the combined alkali burn in vivo-in vitro model. After alkali-induced defect induction, these bulbi were

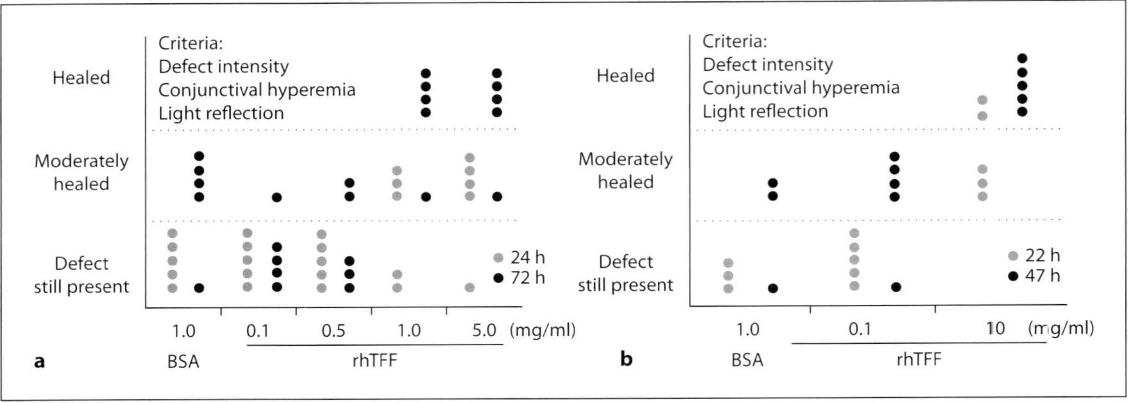

Fig. 3. Topical application of rhTFF3 enhances corneal healing in vivo after alkali-induced and excimer-laser-induced defects. **a** Defects induced by alkaline solution: 5 corneas of each group were treated with rhTFF3 or BSA for 24 or 72 h. **b** Defects induced by excimer laser were allowed to heal in the constant presence of rhTFF3 or BSA for 22 or 47 h. Afterwards, corneas were evaluated according the remaining defect intensity (wound extent and depth), conjunctival hyperemia (signs of inflammation) and light reflection (signs of smoothness of the cornea), and grouped into 3 categories. Results demonstrated the dose-dependent effects of rhTFF3 treatment. From Paulsen et al. [20].

allowed to recover in vitro in the presence of different concentrations of rhTFF3 peptide, BSA or no additives as a control. The healing process was again documented after several time periods. A concentration of 0.1 mg/ml rhTFF3 was found to greatly enhance corneal healing in this model compared to higher concentrations of rhTFF3, BSA or untreated control (fig. 4). Cultivating the bulbi with higher concentrations of the rhTFF3 peptide seems to have no further effect on the recovery of surface integrity compared to BSA. When comparing in vivo and in vivo-in vitro results, it seems obvious that the in vivo model needs higher doses to complete rapid wound closure. However, vital circumstances have to be taken into account as these differences between in vivo and in the combined in vivo-in vitro model might be due to blinking. Parts of the topically applied rhTFF3 might be quickly removed after blinking, so lower doses remain at the ocular surface and ensure rapid re-epithelialization instead of the applied high doses. Moreover, TFF3 results are thought to be receptor-mediated, so a dose-dependent limitation in receptor activation is possible. RhTFF3 treatment with 0.1 mg/ml revealed a quite obvious enhancement in corneal healing in the combined in vivo-in vitro model. These findings correlate with the in vitro studies which found a similar concentration to be most beneficial [35]. Additionally, and even more interestingly, exogenously applied rhTFF3 also produced beneficial effects in $Tff3^{-/-}$ mice. The data are in line with observations in several other animal models of gastrointestinal impairments which show positive effects after TFF3 treatment [14]. Furthermore, a recently published phase-II clinical trial lends weight to this assumption. In the course of that phase-II randomized double-blind placebo-

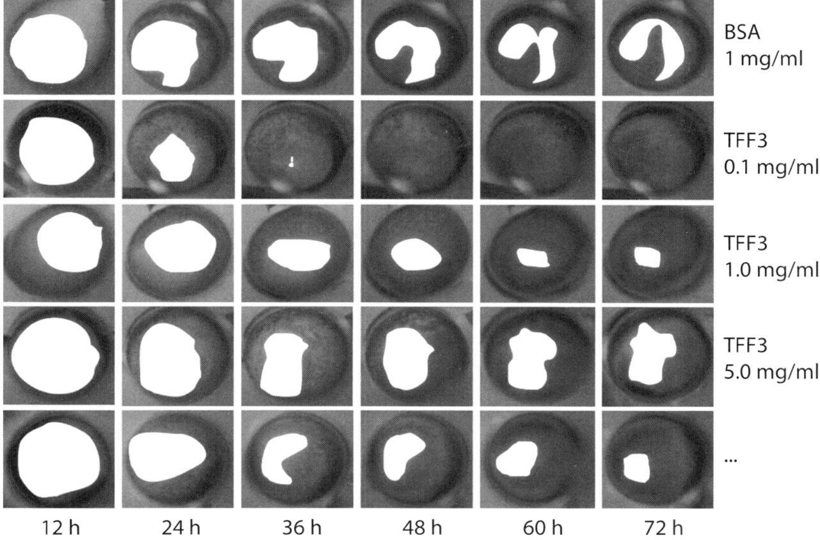

Fig. 4. rhTFF3 enhances corneal healing in an alkali-induced in vivo-in vitro corneal defect model. Alkali-induced defects in each group of 6 corneas were allowed to partially heal in vivo for 6 h, followed by further in vitro cultivation in the presence of rhTFF3, BSA or no additives as a control for up to an additional 72 h. Photographs were taken after 12, 24, 36, 48, 60 and 72 h, and analysis of the wounded area was carried out by measuring the remaining defect area using photo software. For better visualization, corneal defects are marked in white. Treatment with 0.1 mg/ml rhTFF3 led to highly accelerated recovery, whereas increasing concentrations of rhTFF3 had no further effect. From Paulsen et al. [20].

controlled clinical study, rhTFF3 was topically applied as oral spray for prevention of oral mucositis in chemotherapy patients with colorectal cancer. Prophylactic application of both high and low doses of TFF3 produced a reduction in occurrence and severity of oral mucositis compared to the placebo-treated group [41].

Taken together – i.e. inducible expression under pathological conditions, decelerated corneal healing in Tff3$^{-/-}$ mice, beneficial effects of exogenously applied TFF3 on corneal healing in wild-type and Tff3-deficiency mice in corneal defect models, and the positive influence on tear fluid from patients with dry eye syndrome – clinical trial results strengthen the hypothesis that TFF3 is a promising therapeutic candidate for treating corneal injuries, as well as ocular surface impairments caused by dry eye syndrome.

TFF3 in Articular Cartilage

Following the promise offered by TFF3, Rösler et al. [42] conducted studies in articular cartilage since this shares characteristics with the cornea. Both tissues are nonvascular and pathological conditions, such as the main form of dry eye syndrome and osteoarthritis, are to some extent alike in the course of inflammatory progress and the resulting consequences. Osteoarthritis is a degenerative disease characterized by chronic inflammatory conditions. It has a relatively high incidence in Germany, and 25% of 50-year-olds and 80% of 75-year-olds show radiologically visible signs of osteoarthritis. In the course of the chronic inflammatory process, release of proinflammatory cytokines (in particular IL-1β and TNF-α) results in an elevated activation of extracellular matrix-degrading matrix metalloproteinases (MMPs). The inhibitors of the MMPs (tissue inhibitors of matrix metalloproteinases; TIMPs) are downregulated in osteoarthritis, leading to progressive degradation of the extracellular matrix and cartilage [43, 44].

To study the endogenous expression pattern of TFF3, healthy and osteoarthritic articular cartilage was evaluated first. Similar to the findings in the cornea [19], TFF3 expression was only induced under pathological conditions in tissue obtained from osteoarthritic cartilage, whereas in healthy tissue no TFF3 was present. In vivo models like STR/Ort mice (a model for osteoarthritis) also mirrored induced Tff3 expression. This is similar to the observation of emerging Tff3 in murine knee joints of Balb/c mice after injection of bacterial supernatants to simulate septic arthritis, which may also contribute to its role in immune response. Primary chondrocytes obtained from osteoarthritic joints already expressed TFF3 in vitro on a low basal level; however, stimulation with the proinflammatory cytokines IL-1β and TNF-α (two of the key regulators of osteoarthritis) also strongly induced TFF3 expression. Subsequent in vitro experiments analyzing the role of these primary chondrocytes in apoptosis revealed a proapoptotic potential of rhTFF3 alone and in combination with TNF-α – a result completely against expectations. Apart from this, expression of MMPs and TIMPs that play a role in osteoarthritis by participating in articular cartilage metabolism and remodeling was altered after exposure to rhTFF3 as well. In a dose-dependent manner, protein levels greatly increased for MMP3 and MMP1, yet only moderately for MMP13 in primary chondrocytes. However, TIMP1 expression was downregulated after rhTFF3 exposure, reflecting extracellular matrix degradation. TIMP2 expression was not affected in primary chondrocytes, but was reduced in a chondrocyte cell line after high-dose TFF3 stimulation [42].

Surprisingly, all these results obtained in vitro in osteoarthritic primary chondrocytes might reflect a new face of TFF3 under simulated chronic inflammatory conditions. This is very interesting, especially when assuming that the main form of dry eye syndrome is a chronic inflammatory disease. Dry eye syndrome (the main form) is also characterized by increased release of proinflammatory cytokines [45–48] and a hyperosmolar tear film [1, 49] leading to activation of MMPs, in particular MMP-9, 1 and 13, and increased apoptosis [50]. Several mouse models simulating dry eye conditions show overexpression of MMPs and apoptosis-associated markers [51–53]. Even the canine dry eye model established by inflammation of the tear ducts shows this phenomenon [54].

Taken together, in acute conditions TFF3 seems to play a crucial role in mucosal protection and repair. However, under chronic inflammatory conditions, such as those occurring during osteoarthritis, it seems to bring forth apoptosis as well as extracellular matrix degradation by activation of certain MMPs and inhibition of their inhibitors. Until now, the appraisal of these findings concerning the character of TFF3 remains unclear – whether these new findings resemble the ocular surface under dry eye conditions as well and whether this new face of TFF3 is beneficial or has negative consequences.

Wound healing is a very complex process regulated by a wide range of growth factors: TFF3, cytokines that stimulate proteolytic enzymes and induce apoptosis and matrix/tissue degradation. The latter two occur in order to eliminate tissue compromised by the defect to prevent further damage and to allow re-epithelialization and recovery of the surface integrity. Under chronic conditions, the balance between short degradation and subsequent repair is altered to ongoing tissue degradation and apoptotic conditions. To what extent TFF3-induced apoptosis and matrix degradation reflect normal processes concerning wound healing still remains unclear, but this is an interesting question and needs further elucidation.

Following the assumption that rhTFF3 accelerates apoptosis and matrix degradation under chronic inflammatory conditions at the ocular surface, it may also slow the healing process. Thus, endogenously induced TFF3 produced by the conjunctiva and secreted into the tear film, as well as additional topically applied rhTFF3, would probably worsen the patient's condition. This may have negative consequences on future drug development.

Before designing further studies on humans to evaluate the effect of TFF3 at the ocular surface, we have to extend our knowledge of the TFF3 mechanism at the molecular level. Subsequent studies will clarify whether TFF3 is beneficial in chronic inflammatory conditions and can act as a therapeutic candidate for treating patients with dry eye syndrome as well as ocular surface defects.

Acknowledgement

Supported by GI Company, Framingham, Mass., USA.

References

1 Brewitt H, Zierhut M, Paulsen F: Physiologie des Tränenfilms. Z prakt Augenheilkd 2008;29:31–40.

2 Dry Eye Workshop Study (DEWS) Group: Research in dry eye: report of the research subcommittee of the International Dry Eye Workshop (2007). Ocul Surf 2007;5:1–194.

3 Paulsen F: TFF3 – Ein vielversprechendes Therapeutikum. Augenspiegel 2006;6:16–17.

4 Taupin D, Podolsky DK: Trefoil factors: initiators of mucosal healing. Nat Rev Mol Cell Biol 2003;4:721–732.

5 Hoffmann W: Trefoil factor family (TFF) peptides and chemokine receptors: a promising relationship. J Med Chem. 2009;52:6505–6510.
6 Jagla W, Wiede A, Hinz M, Dietzmann K, Gülicher D, Gerlach KL, Hoffmann W: Secretion of TFF-peptides by human salivary glands. Cell Tissue Res 1999;298:161–166.
7 Wiede A, Hinz M, Canzler E, Franke K, Quednow C, Hoffmann W: Synthesis and localization of the mucin-associated TFF-peptides in the human uterus. Cell Tissue Res 2001;303:109–115.
8 Poulsom R, Hanby AM, Lalani EN, Hauser F, Hoffmann W, Stamp GW: Intestinal trefoil factor (TFF 3) and pS2 (TFF 1), but not spasmolytic polypeptide (TFF 2) mRNAs are co-expressed in normal, hyperplastic, and neoplastic human breast epithelium. J Pathol 1997;183:30–38.
9 Vestergaard EM, Nexo E, Wendt A, Guthmann F: Trefoil factors in human milk. Early Hum Dev 2008; 84:631–635.
10 Wiede A, Jagla W, Welte T, Köhnlein T, Busk H, Hoffmann W: Localization of TFF3, a new mucus-associated peptide of the human respiratory tract. Am J Respir Crit Care Med 1999;159:1330–1335.
11 Jagla W, Wiede A, Dietzmann K, Rutkowski K, Hoffmann W: Co-localization of TFF3 peptide and oxytocin in the human hypothalamus. FASEB J 2000;14:1126–1131.
12 Paulsen F, Varoga D, Paulsen A, Tsokos M: Trefoil factor family (TFF) peptides of normal human Vater's ampulla. Cell Tissue Res 2005;321:67–74.
13 Kouznetsova I, Kalinski T, Peitz U, Mönkemüller KE, Kalbacher H, Vieth M, Meyer F, Roessner A, Malfertheiner P, Lippert H, Hoffmann W: Localization of TFF3 peptide in human esophageal submucosal glands and gastric cardia: differentiation of two types of gastric pit cells along the rostro-caudal axis. Cell Tissue Res 2007;328:365–374.
14 Kjellev S: The trefoil factor family-small peptides with multiple functionalities. Cell Mol Life Sci 2008;66:1350–1369.
15 Langer G, Jagla W, Behrens-Baumann W, Walter S, Hoffmann W: Secretory peptides TFF1 and TFF3 synthesized in human conjunctival goblet cells. Invest Ophthalmol Vis Sci 1999;40:2220–2224.
16 Langer G, Walter S, Behrens-Baumann W, Hoffmann W: TFF-Peptide: neue Mukus-assoziierte Sekretionsprodukte der Konjunktiva. Ophthalmologe 2001;98:976–979.
17 Paulsen F, Hinz M, Schaudig U, Thale A, Hoffmann W: TFF peptides in the human efferent tear ducts. Invest Ophthalmol Vis Sci 2002;43:3359–3364.
18 Paulsen FP, Schaudig U, Fabian A, Ehrich D, Sel S: TFF peptides and mucins are major components of dacryoliths. Graefes Arch Clin Exp Ophthalmol 2006;244:1160–1170.
19 Steven P, Schafer G, Nolle B, Hinz M, Hoffmann W, Paulsen F: Distribution of TFF peptides in corneal disease and pterygium. Peptides 2004;25:819–825.
20 Paulsen FP, Woon CW, Varoga D, Jansen A, Garreis F, Jäger K, Amm M, Podolsky DK, Steven P, Barker NP, Sel S: Intestinal trefoil factor/TFF3 promotes re-epithelialization of corneal wounds. J Biol Chem 2008;283:13418–13427.
21 Otto WR, Thim L: Trefoil factor family-interacting proteins. Cell Mol Life Sci 2005;62:2939–2946.
22 Dubeykovskaya Z, Dubeykovskiy A, Solal-Cohen J, Wang TC: Secreted trefoil factor 2 activates CXCR4 receptor in epithelial and lymphocytic cancer cell lines. J Biol Chem 2009;284:3650–3662.
23 Hoffmann W: Trefoil factor family (TFF) peptides and chemokine receptors: a promising relationship. J Med Chem 2009;52:6505–6510.
24 Tomasetto C, Masson R, Linares JL, Wendling C, Lefebvre O, Chenard MP, Rio MC: pS2/TFF1 interacts directly with the VWFC cysteine-rich domains of mucins. Gastroenterology 2000;118:70–80.
25 Thim L, Madsen F, Poulsen SS: Effect of trefoil factors on the viscoelastic properties of mucus gels. Eur J Clin Invest 2002;32:519–527.
26 Paulsen FP, Berry MS: Mucins and TFF peptides of the tear film and lacrimal apparatus. Prog Histochem Cytochem 2006;41:1–53.
27 Cook GA, Familari M, Thim L, Giraud AS: The trefoil peptides TFF2 and TFF3 are expressed in rat lymphoid tissues and participate in the immune response. FEBS Lett 1999;456:155–159.
28 Baus-Loncar M, Kayademir T, Takaishi S, Wang T: Trefoil factor family 2 deficiency and immune response. Cell Mol Life Sci 2005;62:2947–2955.
29 Leung WK, Yu J, Chan FKL, To KF, Chan MWY, Ebert MPA, Ng EKW, Chung SCS, Malfertheiner P, Sung JJY: Expression of trefoil peptides (TFF1, TFF2, and TFF3) in gastric carcinomas, intestinal metaplasia, and non-neoplastic gastric tissues. J Pathol 2002;197:582–588.
30 Emami S, Rodrigues S, Rodrigue CM, Le Floch N, Rivat C, Attoub S, Bruyneel E, Gespach C: Trefoil factor family (TFF) peptides and cancer progression. Peptides 2004;25:885–898.
31 Kinoshita T, Taupin DR, Itoh H, Podolsky DK: Distinct pathways of cell migration and antiapoptotic response to epithelial injury: structure-function analysis of human intestinal trefoil factor. Mol Cell Biol 2000;20:4680–4690.
32 Chen YH, Lu Y, De Plaen IG, Wang LY, Tan XD: Transcription factor NF-kappaB signals antianoikic function of trefoil factor 3 on intestinal epithelial cells. Biochem Biophys Res Commun 2000;274:576–582.
33 Taupin DR, Kinoshita K, Podolsky DK: Intestinal trefoil factor confers colonic epithelial resistance to apoptosis. Proc Natl Acad Sci USA 2000;97:799–804.

34 LeSimple P, van Seuningen I, Buisine MP, Copin MC, Hinz M, Hoffmann W, Hajj R, Brody SL, Coraux C, Puchelle E: Trefoil factor family 3 peptide promotes human airway epithelial ciliated cell differentiation. Am J Respir Cell Mol Biol 2007;36:296–303.
35 Göke MN, Cook JR, Kunert KS, Fini ME, Gipson IK, Podolsky DK: Trefoil peptides promote restitution of wounded corneal epithelial cells. Exp Cell Res 2001;264:337–344.
36 Oertel M, Graness A, Thim L, Bühling F, Kalbacher H, Hoffmann W: Trefoil factor family-peptides promote migration of human bronchial epithelial cells: synergistic effect with epidermal growth factor. Am J Respir Cell Mol Biol 2001;25:418–424.
37 Dürer U, Hartig R, Bang S, Thim L, Hoffmann W: TFF3 and EGF induce different migration patterns of intestinal epithelial cells in vitro and trigger increased internalization of E-cadherin. Cell Physiol Biochem 2007;20:329–346.
38 Storesund T, Hayashi K, Kolltveit KM, Bryne M, Schenck K: Salivary trefoil factor 3 enhances migration of oral keratinocytes. Eur J Oral Sci 2008;116:135–140.
39 Hoffmann W: Trefoil factors TFF (trefoil factor family) peptide-triggered signals promoting mucosal restitution. Cell Mol Life Sci 2005;62:2932–2938.
40 Mashimo H, Wu DC, Podolsky DK, et al: Impaired defense of intestinal mucosa in mice lacking intestinal trefoil factor. Science 1996;274:262–265.
41 Peterson DE, Barker NP, Akhmadullina LI, Rodionova I, Sherman NZ, Davidenko IS, Rakovskaya GN, Gotovkin EA, Shinkarev SA, Kopp MV, Kulikov EP, Moiseyenko VM, Gertner JM, Firsov I, Tuleneva T, Yarosh A, Woon CW: Phase II, randomized, double-blind, placebo-controlled study of recombinant human intestinal trefoil factor oral spray for prevention of oral mucositis in patients with colorectal cancer who are receiving fluorouracil-based chemotherapy. J Clin Oncol 2009;27:4333–4338.
42 Rösler S, Haase T, Claassen H, Schulze U, Schicht M, Riemann D, Barker NP, Brandt J, Wohlrab D, Müller-Hilke B, Goldring MB, Sel S, Varago D, Garreis F, Paulsen FP: TFF3 is induced during degenerative and inflammatory joint disease, activates MMPs and enhances apoptosis of articular cartilage chondrocytes. Arthritis Rheum 2010, in press.
43 Goldring MB: The role of the chondrocyte in osteoarthritis. Arthritis Rheum 2000;43:1916–1926.
44 Fernandes JC, Martel-Pelletier J, Pelletier JP: The role of cytokines in osteoarthritis pathophysiology. Biorheology 2002;39:237–246.
45 Pflugfelder SC, Solomon A, Stern ME: The diagnosis and management of dry eye: a twenty-five-year review. Cornea 2000;19:644–649.
46 Pflugfelder SC: Antiinflammatory therapy for dry eye. Am J Ophthalmol 2004;137:337–342.
47 Li DQ, Shang TY, Kim HS, Solomon A, Lokeshwar BL, Pflugfelder SC: Regulated expression of collagenases MMP-1, -8, and -13 and stromelysins MMP-3, -10, and -11 by human corneal epithelial cells. Invest Ophthalmol Vis Sci 2003;44:2928–2936.
48 Li DQ, Pflugfelder SC: Matrix metalloproteinases in corneal inflammation. Ocul Surf 2005;3:198–202.
49 Li DQ, Chen Z, Song XJ, Luo L, Pflugfelder SC: Stimulation of matrix metalloproteinases by hyperosmolarity via a JNK pathway in human corneal epithelial cells. Invest Ophthalmol Vis Sci 2004;45:4302–4311.
50 Luo L, Li DQ, Pflugfelder SC: Hyperosmolarity-induced apoptosis in human corneal epithelial cells is mediated by cytochrome c and MAPK pathways. Cornea 2007;26:452–460.
51 Brignole F, Pisella PJ, Goldschild M, De Saint Jean M, Goguel A, Baudouin C: Flow cytometric analysis of inflammatory markers in conjunctival epithelial cells of patients with dry eyes. Invest Ophthalmol Vis Sci 2000;41:1356–1363.
52 Luo L, Li DQ, Doshi A, Farley W, Corrales RM, Pflugfelder SC: Experimental dry eye stimulates production of inflammatory cytokines and MMP-9 and activates MAPK signaling pathways on the ocular surface. Invest Ophthalmol Vis Sci 2004;45:4293–4301.
53 Corrales RM, Stern ME, De Paiva CS, Welch J, Li DQ, Pflugfelder SC: Desiccating stress stimulates expression of matrix metalloproteinases by the corneal epithelium. Invest Ophthalmol Vis Sci 2006;47:3293–3302.
54 Nagelhout TJ, Gamache DA, Roberts L, Brady MT, Yanni JM: Preservation of tear film integrity and inhibition of corneal injury by dexamethasone in a rabbit model of lacrimal gland inflammation-induced dry eye. J Ocul Pharmacol Ther 2005;21:139–148.

Ute Schulze
Department of Anatomy and Cell Biology, Martin Luther University
Grosse Steinstrasse 52
DE–06097 Halle/Saale (Germany)
Tel. +49 345 557 1712, Fax +49 345 557 1700, E-Mail ute.schulze@medizin.uni-halle.de

Brewitt H (ed): Research Projects in Dry Eye Syndrome.
Dev Ophthalmol. Basel, Karger, 2010, vol 45, pp 12–15

Cationic Amino Acid Transporters and β-Defensins in Dry Eye Syndrome

Kristin Jäger · Fabian Garreis · Matthias Dunse · Friedrich P. Paulsen

Department of Anatomy and Cell Biology, Martin Luther University of Halle-Wittenberg, Halle/Saale, Germany

Abstract

Several diseases concomitant with L-arginine deficiency (diabetes, chronic kidney failure, psoriasis) are significantly associated with dry eye syndrome. One important factor that has so far been neglected is the y^+ transporter. In humans, y^+ accounts for nearly 80% of arginine transport, exclusively carrying the cationic amino acids L-arginine, L-lysine and L-ornithine. y^+ is represented by CAT (cationic amino acid transporter) proteins. L-arginine is a precursor of the moisturizer urea, which has been used in the treatment of dry skin diseases. Although urea has also been shown to be part of the tear film, little attention has been paid to it in this role. Moreover, L-arginine and L-lysine are major components contributing to synthesis of the antimicrobially active β-defensins induced under dry eye conditions. The first results have demonstrated that transport of L-arginine and L-lysine into epithelial cells is limited by the y^+ transporter at the ocular surface.

Fifty-five million ocular injuries occur each year worldwide [1]. Recent studies have shown that one third of all 4-year-olds exhibit deficiencies in visual acuity, of which only 40% are recognized. These deficiencies can be traced in part to previous ocular infections [2]. In the majority of cases, irreversible long-term damage can be expected due to late recognition of the problem. The correction of refractive errors is common today, and as a result approximately 30 million people in Germany wear glasses or contact lenses, with the figure in the USA reaching about 120 million. Wearing poorly adjusted or inadequately cleaned contact lenses increases the risk of inflammation of the ocular surface considerably [3–5]. Over the last few years and with increasing frequency, refractive errors have been corrected using laser-assisted in situ keratomileusis (LASIK). Thus, by the year 2000, about 1.55 million operations had already been reported in the USA. The frequency of laser treatment is growing worldwide by about 10–25% per year. Although LASIK is considered to be safer and less prone to complications than photorefractive keratectomy and radial keratectomy, problems with secondary infections arise here as well, as is the case in all ocular operations [6, 7].

In general, bacterial keratitis and conjunctivitis are the most common diagnoses in ophthalmological practice. They most frequently appear subsequent to long-term contact lens use, refractive corneal surgery, penetrating corneal injury and in the course of immunosuppressive treatment [8–11]. The most common pathogens found to induce keratitis are *Staphylococcus aureus* and *Pseudomonas aeruginosa* [12, 13]. The bacterial products of metabolism and their toxins as well as the inflammatory reaction of the host often result in severe tissue injury with lasting scarring, potentially leading to complete loss of vision [8].

Functional Relationship between y^+ Transporter and β-Defensins

The ocular surface, constantly exposed to environmental pathogens, is particularly vulnerable to infection. An advanced immune defense system is therefore essential to protect the eye from microbial attack. Antimicrobial peptides, such as β-defensins, are essential components of the innate immune system and are the first line of defense against invaders. In order to produce defensins, the cells forming them require large amounts of the amino acids L-arginine and L-lysine. In humans, the amino acids are transferred through the cell membrane via the y^+ transporter approximately 80% of the time. The remaining 20% are transported non-specifically via the transporters $B^{0,+}$, $b^{0,+}$ and y^{+-L}, which play only a minor role in L-arginine and L-lysine transport and, up to now, no role at all in the immune response [14]. An inadequate supply of the cationic amino acids L-lysine and L-arginine, secondary to a blockage or destruction of the cationic amino acid transporters, could lead to reduction or cessation of β-defensin production. In particular, production of the defensins (human β-defensin; hBD-2 and 3) could be affected, the expressions of which are induced by various cytokines or bacterial toxins. Experiments on cationic amino acid transporter knockout ($CAT2^{-/-}$) mouse mutants have shown NO production to decrease by 95% and L-arginine uptake by 92% in inflammation [15]. There is thus a direct consequence of $CAT2^{-/-}$. Such an effect is presumably related to hBD-2 and/or 3 production.

hBD-2 was first obtained from psoriatic skin. It has been demonstrated that psoriasis patients have fewer dermal infections than would be expected from the condition of the skin. This led to speculation that psoriatic skin lesions may produce antimicrobial peptides that protect it from infection [16]. It is also known that psoriatic skin or dry skin per se is always accompanied by urea deficiency. Urea is formed in the breakdown process of specific amino acids, particularly arginine, in the keratinization process of the cells. In keratinization disturbances, there is a lack of these amino acids, especially arginine. This leads to a clear reduction in urea concentration, and the natural moisture-retaining function is reduced. In comparative measurements, urea concentrations reduced by as much as 50% were found in clinically dry skin as compared to healthy skin [17]. This lack of natural moisture-retaining factors (particularly urea) leads to increased transepidermal water loss. The skin becomes dry and open lesions develop in the epidermis.

Generally, in diseases accompanied by L-arginine deficiency [18, 19], e.g. psoriasis, dry skin, diabetes or rheumatoid arthritis, there is a significant association with dry eye [20] as well as increased β-defensin production [21]. Although the details of these relationships have been known for some time, to date their interrelatedness has not been considered.

Research Project

For the first time, our group succeeded in localizing the y^+ transporter in form of hCAT1 and hCAT2 in tissues of the ocular surface and lacrimal apparatus. Moreover, we were able to demonstrate that changes in hCAT expression occur during specific corneal diseases and through inflammatory mediators [22]. Our own investigations had established the relationship between the y^+ transporter and psoriasis [19, 23], and the relationship between β-defensins and pathological changes at the ocular surface was established [24]. We now have initial evidence of a direct correlation between dermatoses related to dry skin and dry eye syndrome. With regard to this, a questionnaire-based study revealed that 63% of patients (n >300) with diagnosed dry eye also suffer from dry skin (unpublished results). These results and the current literature support the assumption that the y^+ transporter is involved in dry eye pathology. The current project therefore aims to analyze whether the y^+ transporter is involved in a causal regulation cascade of β-defensins, urea and dry eye syndrome, with the prospect of opening up new avenues in treatment of dry eyes.

References

1 WHO: Program for the Prevention of Blindness, 2004.

2 Federal Association of Ophthalmologists: Communication of the (German) Federal Association of Ophthalmologists, 2006.

3 Ky W, Scherick K, Stenson S: Clinical survey of lens in contact lens patients. CLAO J 1998;24:216–219.

4 Choy MH, Stapleton F, Willcox MD, Zhu H: Comparison of virulence factors in *Pseudomonas aeruginosa* strains isolated from contact lens- and non-contact lens-related keratitis. J Med Microbiol 2008;57(part 12):1539–1546.

5 Rau G, Seedor JA, Shah MK, Ritterband DC, Koplin RS: Incidence and clinical characteristics of *Enterococcus* keratitis. Cornea 2008;27:895–899.

6 Freitas D, Alvarenga L, Sampaio J, Mannis M, Sato E, Sousa L, Vieira L, Yu MC, Martins MC, Hoffling-Lima A, Belfort R Jr: An outbreak of *Mycobacterium chelonae* infection after LASIK. Ophthalmology 2003;110:276–285.

7 Garg P, Bansal AK, Sharma S, Vemuganti GK: Bilateral infectious keratitis after laser in situ keratomileusis: a case report and review of the literature. Ophthalmology. 2001;108:121–125.

8 Baum J: Infection of the eye. Clin Infect Dis 1995;21: 479–488.

9 Gritz DC, Whitcher JP: Topical issues in the treatment of bacterial keratitis. Int Ophthalmol Clin 1998;38:107–114.

10 Brennan NA, Chantal Coles ML: Extended wear in perspective. Invest Ophthalmol Vis Sci 1997;74:609–623.

11 Levartovsky S, Rosenwasser G, Goodman D: Bacterial keratitis following laser in situ keratomileusis. Ophthalmology 2001;108:321–325.
12 Fleisig SMJ, Efron N, Pier GB: Extended contact lens wear enhances *Pseudomonas aeruginosa* adherence to human corneal epithelium. Invest Ophthalmol Vis Sci 1992;33:2908–2916.
13 O'Callaghan RJ, Cellegan MC, Moreau JM, Green LC, Foster TJ, Hartford OM, Engel LS, Hill JM: Specific roles of alpha-toxin and beta-toxin during *Staphylococcus aureus* corneal infection. Infect Immun 1997; 65:1571–1578.
14 Deves R, Boyd CAR: Transporters for cationic amino acids in animal cells: discovery, structure, and function. Physiol Rev 1998;78:478–545.
15 Nicholson B, Manner CK, Kleeman J, MacLeod CL: Sustained nitric oxide production in macrophages requires the arginine transporter CAT2. J Biol Chem 2001;276:15881–15885.
16 Harder J, Bartels J, Christophers E, Schröder JM: A peptide antibiotic from human skin. Nature 1997; 387:861.
17 Wellner K, Fiedler G, Wohlrab W: Untersuchungen zum Harnstoffgehalt der Hornschicht bei Neurodermitis. Z Hautkr 1992;67:648–650.
18 Lucotti P, Setola E, Monti LD, Galluccio E, Costa S, Sandoli EP, Fermo I, Rabaiotti G, Gatti R, Piatti P: Beneficial effects of a long-term oral L-arginine treatment added to a hypocaloric diet and exercise training program in obese, insulin-resistant type 2 diabetic patients. Am J Physiol Endocrinol Metab 2006;291:906–912.
19 Jaeger K, Paulsen F, Wohlrab J: Characterization of cationic amino acid transporters (hCATs) 1 and 2 in human skin. Histochem Cell Biol 2008;129:321–329.
20 Rahman A, Yahya K, Ahmed T, Sharif-Ul-Hasan K: Diagnostic value of tear films tests in type 2 diabetes. J Pak Med Assoc. 2007;57:577–581.
21 McDermot AM: Defensins and other antimicrobial peptides at the ocular surface. Ocul Surf 2004;2:229–247.
22 Jaeger K, Boenisch U, Risch M, Worlitzsch D, Paulsen FP: Detection of cationic amino acid transporters in the human lacrimal system and their involvement in ocular surface disease. Invest Ophthalmol Vis Sci 2009;50:1112–1121.
23 Recker K, Klapperstück T, Kehlen A, Wohlrab J: The Importance of Cationic Amino Acid Transporter Expression in Human Skin. J Invest Dermatol 2003;121:1552–1553.
24 Garreis F, Schlorf T, Worlitzsch D, Steven P, Bräuer L, Jäger K, Paulsen F: Roles of human ß-defensins in innate immune defense at the ocular surface: arming and alarming corneal and conjunctival epithelial cells. Exp Eye Res 2010, submitted.

Dr. rer. nat. Kristin Jäger
Department of Anatomy and Cell Biology, Martin Luther University of Halle-Wittenberg
Grosse Steinstrasse 52
DE–06097 Halle/Saale (Germany)
Tel. +49 345 557 1740, Fax +49 345 557 1700, E-Mail kristin.jaeger@medizin.uni-halle.de

Brewitt H (ed): Research Projects in Dry Eye Syndrome.
Dev Ophthalmol. Basel, Karger, 2010, vol 45, pp 16–22

Antimicrobial Peptides as a Major Part of the Innate Immune Defense at the Ocular Surface

Fabian Garreis · Maria Gottschalt · Friedrich P. Paulsen

Department of Anatomy and Cell Biology, Martin Luther University Halle-Wittenberg, Halle/Saale, Germany

Abstract

The ocular surface is in constant contact with the environment (e.g. when using one's fingers to insert a contact lens) and thus also with diverse bacteria, bacterial components and their pathogen-associated molecules. Dysfunctions of the tear film structure or decreased moistening of the ocular surface, as in dry eye (keratoconjunctivitis sicca) for example, often lead to inflammatory and infectious complications resulting in severe functional disorders, particularly concerning the cornea. Besides different protective antimicrobial substances in the tear fluid (mucins, lysozyme, lactoferrin), the epithelia of cornea and conjunctiva can also protect themselves from microbial invasion by producing an arsenal of antimicrobial peptides (AMPs). A number of different studies have revealed that small cationic AMPs, which display antimicrobial activity against a broad spectrum of microorganisms, are a major component of the innate immune system at the human ocular surface. Furthermore, several AMPs modulate cellular activation processes like migration, proliferation, chemotaxis and cytokine production, and in this way also affect the adaptive immune system. In this article, we have summarized current knowledge of the mechanisms of activity and functional roles of AMPs, with a focus on potential multifunctional roles of human β-defensins and S100 peptide psoriasin (S100A7) at the ocular surface.

Antimicrobial Peptides at the Ocular Surface

Lacrimation and the wiper function of the eyelids are effective in counteracting invasion and colonization of microorganisms at the ocular surface. Additionally, the tear film contains a number of unspecific antibacterial substances, like lysozyme, lactoferrin, lipocalins, secretory phospholipase A_2 and components of the complement system [1]. Another primary defense mechanism of the innate immune system involves antimicrobial peptides (AMPs). AMPs are defined as peptide molecules which show direct antimicrobial activity, are less than 100 amino acids in length and are coded by individual genes. Moreover, due to the high amount of cationic amino acids, AMPs have a positive net charge in physiological pH conditions and their structure is characterized by a hydrophobic and a hydrophilous side (amphipathic character). AMPs have been detected across a wide spectrum of different species, including amoeba, plants, insects and mammals. A database maintained by the University of Trieste (www.bbcm.units.it/~tossi/pag1.htm) contains a list of over 900 AMPs and proteins. They are classified into 4 groups according to their secondary structure: (1) linear α-helical peptides (e.g. human cathelicidin LL-37); (2) peptides with β-sheets and disulfide bonds (e.g. α- and β-defensins); (3) peptides with a high amount of specific amino acids (e.g. histatin family); (4) peptides with a loop domain (e.g. bactenecin) [2–4]. The major AMPs present at the ocular surface are α- and β-defensins and human cathelicidin LL-37, also a number of others have been identified at the ocular surface (fig. 1). These AMPs have been detected in cells from the lacrimal gland, glands of Krause and Moll, and also from cornea and conjunctiva epithelia [for a review, see 5].

AMP Active Principle

AMPs demonstrate direct antimicrobial activity against a broad spectrum of Gram-positive and Gram-negative bacteria, fungi and some viruses. Antibacterial activity occurs in a low micromolar range, and AMPs show large variability in their efficiency in killing specific pathogens. The active principle of AMPs, namely the direct antimicrobial activity, is based on the charge-dependent interaction of the positively charged AMPs with the negatively charged surface of microorganisms. The detailed mechanism of the electrostatic interaction, however, is still being researched and discussed at the moment [6], but all models show permeabilization of the microbial cell membrane, which leads to loss of essential intracellular components and cell death. Furthermore, several alternative mechanisms of AMP activity have also been described, which contain partly specific interactions with receptor molecules or intracellular molecules. Current studies also show that AMPs take up important mammalian functions concerning cellular activation processes (like proliferation, migration, chemotaxis and cytokine production [7, 8]) and linking the innate with the adaptive immune system [9–11].

AMPs and Dry Eye

Dry eye disease (keratoconjunctivitis sicca) is one of the most frequent chronic diseases of the ocular surface worldwide. Here, all symptoms are subsumed, causing decreased moistening of the ocular surface with tear fluid (DEWS report 2007). This is due to a wide range of environmental factors (screen work, air conditioning), but also numerous general and systemic diseases (Sjogren's syndrome, diabetes mellitus, rheumatic diseases). From a clinical view, it is known that patients with sicca syndrome are more

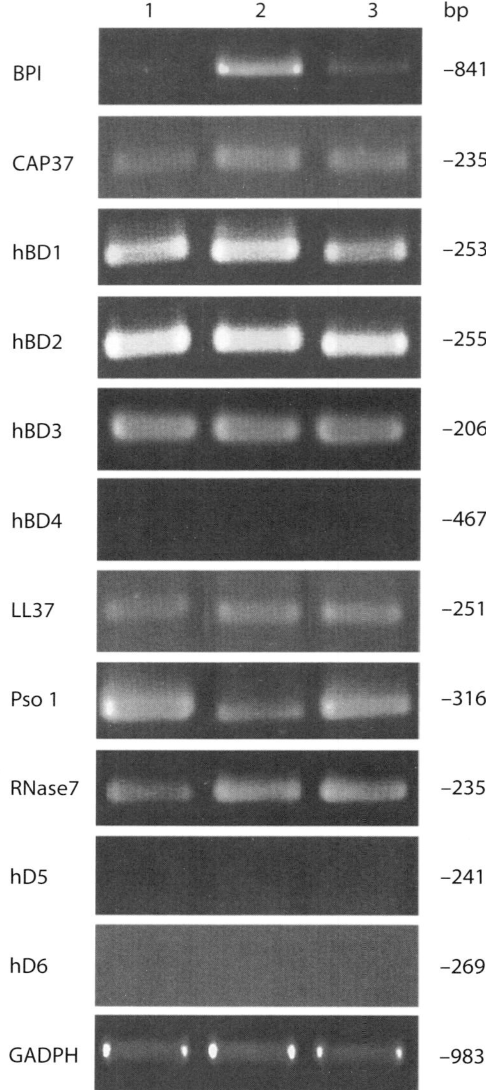

Fig. 1. AMP expression in human conjunctival epithelium. RT-PCR was performed using RNA isolated from the conjunctiva of 3 different cadavers (ethidium bromide-stained 1% agarose gels). All samples expressed bactericidal permeability-increasing protein (BPI), heparin-binding protein (CAP37), human β-defensin (hBD1, 2 and 3), human cathelicidin (LL-37), psoriasin (Pso 1) and RNase7. No expression could be detected from hBD4 or human defensin 5 or 6 (HD5, HD6) in human conjunctival epithelial cells. To estimate correlations, a GAPDH PCR was performed for each tissue investigated.

susceptible to infectious diseases of the eye [12, 13]. On the one hand, it has been shown that patients with dry eye have decreased secretion of certain antibacterial substances (lysozyme, lactoferrin) into the tear fluid [14]. On the other hand, it has been proven that human β-defensin (hBD) 2 is upregulated in mild forms of dry eye [15]. Moreover, some studies have shown that β-defensins activate dendritic and T cells, which are involved in initiating the inflammatory reaction seen in dry eye [16–18].

In the tear fluid, there are different constitutively produced and inducible AMPs. These AMPs are produced by different cells of the lacrimal gland, accessory lacrimal glands, and corneal and conjunctival epithelia, and they are secreted into the tear fluid. An excerpt from our own research on AMPs at the ocular surface has been summarized later in this report.

Human β-Defensins

The two major categories of mammalian AMPs at the ocular surface are the defensins and cathelicidins (LL-37) [6]. Defensins are small in size (29–45 amino acids), cationic, and are characterized by the presence of 6 conserved cysteine residues [19]. Based on the distribution of the cysteines and the linkage of disulfide bonds, defensins are classified into 3 subfamilies, referred to as α, β and θ (also minidefensins). In humans, six α-defensins have been identified and characterized in particularly high concentrations in neutrophils (human neutrophil peptides 1–4) [20, 21], intestinal Paneth cells and the female reproductive tract (human defensins 5 and 6) [22–24]. The α-defensins are expressed constitutively and matured peptides are stored in cell granules. The first characterized hBD1–3 are primarily produced by keratinocytes, mucosal epithelial cells of various tissues, and immune cells (such as monocytes, dendritic cells and macrophages) [25]. hBD4 is found in the testis and uterus, and expressions of hBD5 and 6 are restricted to the epididymis [26]. θ-Defensins are not translated in humans due to premature stop codons [27].

At the ocular surface, α-defensins have been detected in infiltrating neutrophils, and production and secretion by ocular surface epithelial cells has also been shown [6]. Zhou et al. [28] detected the presence of human neutrophil peptides 1–3 in tear film (0.2–1 μg/ml) using liquid chromatography mass spectrometry; no evidence of human defensin 5 or 6 production was found. Corneal and conjunctival epithelial cells are bathed in tears that contain low concentrations of neutrophil defensins in normal (open eye) conditions and become elevated after surgery [29]. Also, human β-defensins have been shown to be expressed in ocular surface epithelial cells in several studies, including our own. At the ocular surface, hBD1 is constitutively expressed, whereas the expression of hBD2 is variable and inducible by exposure to bacteria, bacterial products (such as lipopolysaccharide and peptidoglycan) and proinflammatory cytokines. Expression of hBD2 is also upregulated in the cornea in response to injury [30] and in the conjunctivial epithelial cells of patient with dry eye [15, 31]. Data obtained in our group demonstrated that in a murine corneal scratch model, mouse β-defensins are only induced if microbial products within the tear film come into contact with a defective epithelium [32]. Corneal and conjunctival cells also express hBD3 on the mRNA and protein levels. hBD3 was shown to have broad-spectrum antimicrobial activity that is less salt-sensitive than other defensins located at the ocular surface [33]. Some studies have indicated that expression of this defensin is inducible by TNF-α and interferon-γ [34, 35]. We have shown that proinflammatory cytokines (IL-1β and TNF-α) and supernatants of Gram-positive bacteria *Staphylococcus aureus* increased the relative expression of the hBD3 transcript and led to the induction of hBD3 peptide secretion in cultivated human corneal epithelial cells (unpublished data). However, β-defensins have also attracted much attention. Several studies, including our own work, have recently suggested that they are multifunctional peptides which also have a multitude of non-antimicrobial functions, such as cell proliferation and death, wound healing, extracellular matrix remodeling [36], cell migration, or functions related to pigmentation (hair color) [37] and feeding behavior among several others [for further details, see 5, 38]. Moreover, abnormal β-defensin expression is associated with inflammatory diseases, such as psoriasis, atopic dermatitis, Crohn's disease and cystic fibrosis [39], and overexpression has been shown to induce progressive muscle degeneration in mice [40]. The functional impact of β-defensins at the ocular surface is further questionable as the effect of physiological salt concentrations in human tears on β-defensin activity revealed a marked reduction or even a loss at low peptide concentrations. Furthermore, we are currently investigating regulation of human β-defensins among each other and their interaction with other proteins of the human tear film (mucins, TFF peptides and surfactant proteins).

Psoriasin and Angiogenin

In our own preliminary examinations, we focused on the significance of the AMPs psoriasin and angiogenin, which are, as of yet, largely unknown at the ocular surface. So, the group of Sack et al. [42] was able to prove using a protein array technique that angiogenin can be found at a much higher concentration in the tear film than many other peptides [42]. We first detected angiogenin in the epithelial cells of human conjunctiva and in the high columnar epithelial cells of the nasolacrimal duct using immunohistochemistry (unpublished data). No expression could be detected in human lacrimal gland or cornea. Gläser et al. [43] first described psoriasin, originally isolated as an overexpressed molecule of unknown function in psoriasis, and has recently been identified as a principal *Escherichia-coli*-killing AMP of healthy skin. Our own RT-PCR and Western blot analyses [44] revealed a constitutive expression of psoriasin in the cornea, conjunctiva and nasolacrimal ducts, but not in the human lacrimal gland. Immunohistochemistry revealed strong staining of meibomian glands for psoriasin and somewhat weaker immunoreactivity in the epithelium of conjunctiva and around the hair follicles of the eyelid. No induction of psoriasin was observed after stimulation with supernatants of *E. coli*, whereas supernatants of *Staphylococcus aureus* and *Haemophilus influenzae* significantly increased the psoriasin mRNA and protein expression. Stimulation with IL-1β and VEGF also strongly increased the psoriasin transcription (unpublished data). The highest amounts of psoriasin were detected in tear fluid of healthy volunteers by means of ELISA experiments. Currently, there are several investigations underway into the regulation of psoriasin and angiogenin at the ocular surface in our research group.

Outlook

The results confirm the key role of AMPs, particularly human β-defensins, in innate immune defense at the ocular surface. Furthermore, the relevance of AMPs psoriasin and angiogenin (largely unknown at the ocular surface) is to be investigated, as is the impact of different stimulants (bacterial components, proinflammatory cytokines, anoxemia, ultraviolet rays) on the production and regulation of AMPs. The results will contribute to the understanding of different reactions and diseases at the ocular surface and, moreover, to the general understanding of the production and regulation of AMPs at the ocular surface and lacrimal apparatus. They will also open up new perspectives for the therapeutical use of recombinant AMPs at the ocular surface, particularly in patients with dry eye.

References

1 Sack RA, Nunes I, Beaton A, Morris C: Host-defense mechanism of the ocular surfaces. Biosci Rep 2001;21:463–480.

2 Bals R: Epithelial antimicrobial peptides in host defense against infection. Respir Res 2000;1:141–150.

3 van't Hof W, Veerman ECI, Helmerhorst EJ, Amerongen AVN: Antimicrobial peptides: properties and applicability. Biol Chem 2001;382:597–619.

4 Boman HG: Antimicrobial peptides: basic facts and emerging concepts. J Intern Med 2003;254:197–215.

5 Paulsen F, Varoga D, Steven P, Pufe T: Antimicrobial peptides at the ocular surface; in Zierhut M, Stern ME, Sullivan DA (eds): Immunology of Lacrimal Gland and Tear Film. London, Taylor & Francis, 2005, pp 97–104.

6 McDermott AM: The role of antimicrobial peptides at the ocular surface. Ophthal Res 2009;41:60–75.

7 Scott MG, Hancock REW: Cationic antimicrobial peptides and their multifunctional role in the immune system. Crit Rev Immunol 2000;20:407–431.

8 Bals R, Wilson JM: Cathelicidins – a family of multifunctional antimicrobial peptides. Cell Mol Life Sci 2003;60:711–720.

9 Yang D, Chertov O, Oppenheim JJ: The role of mammalian antimicrobial peptides and proteins in awakening of innate host defenses and adaptive immunity. Cell Mol Life Sci 2001;58:978–989.

10 Yang D, Biragyn A, Kwak LW, Oppenheim JJ: Mammalian defensins in immunity: more than just antimicrobicidal. Trends Immunol 2002;23:291–296.

11 Yang D, Biragyn A, Hoover DM: Multiple roles of antimicrobial defensins, cathelicidins and eosinophil-derived neurotoxin in host defense. Annu Rev Immunol 2004;22:181–215.

12 Hemady R, Chu W, Foster CS: Keratoconjunctivitis sicca and corneal ulcers. Cornea 1990;9:170–173.

13 Lemp MA, Gold JB: Tear film diagnosis in contact lens wearers (in German). Klin Monatsbl Augenheilkd 1990;197:202–206.

14 McCollum CJ, Foulks GN, Bodner B: Rapid assay of lactoferrin in keratoconjunctivitis sicca. Cornea 1994;13:505–508.

15 Narayanan S, Miller WL, McDermott AM: Expression of human beta-defensins in conjunctival epithelium: relevance to dry eye disease. Invest Ophthalmol Vis Sci 2003;44:3795–3801.

16 Chertov O, Michiel DF, Xu L: Identification of defensin-1, defensin-2, and CAP37/azurocidin as T-cell chemoattractant proteins released from interleukin-8-stimulated neutrophils. J Biol Chem 1996;271:2935–2940.

17 Yang D, Chen Q, Chertov O, Oppenheim JJ: Human neutrophil defensins selectively chemoattract naive T and immature dendritic cells. J Leukoc Biol 2000;68:9–14.

18 Yang D, Chertov O, Bykovskaia SN: Beta-defensins: linking innate and adaptive immunity through dendritic and T cell CCR6. Science 1999;286:525–528.

19 Bowdish DM, Davidson DJ, Hancock RE: Immunomodulatory properties of defensins and cathelicidins. Curr Top Microbiol Immunol 2006;306:27–66.

20 Ganz T, Selsted ME, Szklarek D: Defensins: natural peptide antibiotics of human neutrophils. J Clin Invest 1985;76:1427–1435.

21 Wilde CG, Griffith JE, Marra MN: Purification and characterization of human neutrophil peptide 4, a novel member of the defensin family. J Biol Chem 1989;264:11200–11203.

22 Jones DE, Bevins CL: Paneth cells of the human small intestine express an antimicrobial gene. J Biol Chem 1992;267:23216–23225.
23 Jones DE, Bevins CL: Defensin-6 mRNA in human Paneth cells: implications for antimicrobial peptides in host defense of human bowel. FEBS Lett 1993;315: 187–192.
24 Quayle AJ, Porter EM, Nussbaum AA: Gene expression, immunolocalization and secretion of human defensin-5 in female reproductive tract. Am J Pathol 1998 152:1247–1258.
25 Schneider JJ, Unholzer A, Schaller M, Schäfer-Korting M, Korting HC: Human defensins. J Mol Med 2005;83:587–595.
26 Yang D, Liu ZH, Tewary P, Chen Q, de la Rosa G, Oppenheim JJ: Defensin participation in innate and adaptive immunity. Curr Pharm Des 2007;13:3131–3139.
27 Nguyen TX, Cole AM, Lehrer RI: Evolution of primate theta-defensins: a serpentine path to a sweet tooth. Peptides 2003;24:1647–1654.
28 Zhou L, Huang LQ, Beuerman RW, Grigg ME, Li SF, Chew FT, Ang L, Stern ME, Tan D: Proteomic analysis of human tears: defensin expression after ocular surface surgery. J Proteome Res 2004;3:410–416.
29 McDermott AM, Redfern RL, Zhang B: Human β-defensin 2 is up-regulated during re-epithelialization of the cornea. Curr Eye Res 2001;22:64–67.
30 Kawasaki S, Kawamoto S, Yokoi N, Connon C, Minesaki Y, Kinoshita S, Okubo K: Up-regulated gene expression in the conjunctival epithelium of patients with Sjögren's syndrome. Exp Eye Res 2003; 77:17–26.
31 Garreis F, Schlorf T, Varoga D, Paulsen FP: Ocular surface expression and regulation of β-defensins. Poster 5th Int Tear Film Ocular Surf Conf, Taormina, 2007.
32 Varoga D, Pufe T, Mentlein R: Expression and regulation of antimicrobial peptides in articular joints. Ann Anat 2005;187:499–508.
33 Huang LC, Jean D, Proske RJ, Reins RY, McDermott AM: Ocular surface expression and in vitro activity of antimicrobial peptides. Curr Eye Res 2007;32:595–609.
34 Harder J, Bartels J, Christophers E, Schröder JM: Isolation and characterization of human-beta-defensin-3, a novel inducible peptide antibiotic. J Biol Chem 2001;276:5707–5713.
35 Garcia JR, Jaumann F, Schulz S, Krause A, Rodriguez-Jimenez J, Forssmann U, Adermann K, Kluver E, Vogelmeier C, Becker D, Hedrich R, Forssmann WG, Bals R: Identification of a novel, multifunctional beta-defensin (human beta defensin 3) with specific antimicrobial activity: its interaction with plasma membranes of *Xenopus* oocytes and the induction of macrophage chemoattraction. Cell Tissue Res 2001 306:257–264.
36 Varoga D, Pufe T, Mentlein R, Kohrs S, Grohmann S, Tillmann B, Hassenpflug J, Paulsen F: Expression and regulation of antimicrobial peptides in articular joints. Ann Anat 2005;187:499–508.
37 Candille SI, Kaelin CB, Cattanach BM, Yu B, Thompson DA, Nix MA, Kerns JA, Schmutz SM, Millhauser GL, Barsh GS: A-defensin mutation causes black coat color in domestic dogs. Science 2007;318:1418–1423.
38 Beisswenger C, Bals R: Functions of antimicrobial peptides in host defense and immunity. Curr Protein Pept Sci 2005;6:255–264.
39 Zaiou M: Multifunctional antimicrobial peptides: therapeutic targets in several human diseases. J Mol Med 2007;85:317–329.
40 Yamaguchi Y, Nagase T, Tomita T, Nakamura K, Fukuhara S, Amano T, Yamamoto H, Ide Y, Suzuki M, Teramoto S, Asano T, Kangawa K, Nakagata N, Ouchi Y, Kurihara H: Beta-defensin overexpression induces progressive muscle degeneration in mice. Am J Physiol Cell Physiol 2007;292:C2141–C2149.
41 Hooper LV, Stappenbeck TS, Hong CV, Gordon JI: Angiogenins: a new class of microbicidal proteins involved in innate immunity. Nat Immunol 2003;4: 269–273.
42 Sack RA, Conradi L, Krumholz D, Beaton A, Sathe S, Morris C: Membrane array characterization of 80 chemokines, cytokines, and growth factors in open- and closed-eye tears: angiogenin and other defense system constituents. Invest Ophthalmol Vis Sci 2005;45:1228–1238.
43 Gläser R, Harder J, Lange H, Bartels J, Christophers E, Schröder JM: Antimicrobial psoriasin (S100A7) protects human skin from *Escherichia coli* infection. Nat Immunol 2005;6:57–64.
44 Garreis F, Gottschalt M, Gläser R, Harder J, Worlitzsch D, Paulsen FP: Expression and regulation of antimicrobial peptide psoriasin (S100A7) in the lacrimal apparatus. Poster ARVO Ann Meet, Fort Lauderdale, 2009, No. 5515/A486.

Fabian Garreis
Department of Anatomy and Cell Biology, Martin Luther University Halle-Wittenberg
Grosse Steinstrasse 52
DE–06097 Halle/Saale (Germany)
Tel. +49 345 557 1712, Fax +49 345 557 1700, E-Mail fabian.garreis@medizin.uni-halle.de

Brewitt H (ed): Research Projects in Dry Eye Syndrome.
Dev Ophthalmol. Basel, Karger, 2010, vol 45, pp 23–39

Regulation of the Inflammatory Component in Chronic Dry Eye Disease by the Eye-Associated Lymphoid Tissue (EALT)

Nadja Knop[a] · Erich Knop[b]

[a]Department of Cell Biology in Anatomy, Hannover Medical School, Hannover, and
[b]Research Laboratory, Department of Ophthalmology CVK, Charité – Universitätsmedizin Berlin, Berlin, Germany

Abstract

Purpose: The physiologically protective mucosal immune system of the ocular surface consists of lymphocytes, accessory leukocytes and soluble immune modulators. Their involvement has also been observed in inflammatory ocular surface diseases, including dry eye syndrome, and we have attempted here to describe their interaction. **Methods:** Our own results regarding the mucosal immune system of the human ocular surface are discussed together with the available literature on mucosal immunity and inflammatory ocular surface disease. **Results:** The mucosa of the ocular surface proper (conjunctiva and cornea) is anatomically continuous with its mucosal adnexa (the lacrimal gland and lacrimal drainage system) and contains a mucosal immune system termed 'eye-associated lymphoid tissue' (EALT). This extends from the periacinar lacrimal-gland-associated lymphoid tissue along the excretory ducts into the conjunctiva-associated lymphoid tissue (CALT) and further into the lacrimal drainage-associated lymphoid tissue (LDALT). EALT consists of continuous diffuse lymphoid effector tissue and of interspersed follicles for effector cell generation in CALT and LDALT. Typical events in ocular surface disease include alteration and activation of epithelial cells with loss of epithelial integrity, production of inflammatory cytokines, and potential presentation of non-pathogenic and self-antigens – leading to a loss of immune tolerance. Events in the deregulation of physiologically protective EALT, resulting vicious circles, and eventual self-propagating immunomodulated inflammatory disease processes are explained, discussed and visualized by schematic drawings. **Conclusion:** Deregulation of EALT can orchestrate a self-propagating inflammatory mucosal disease process if the capacity of natural compensatory factors is overridden and if the disease is not limited by timely diagnosis and therapy.

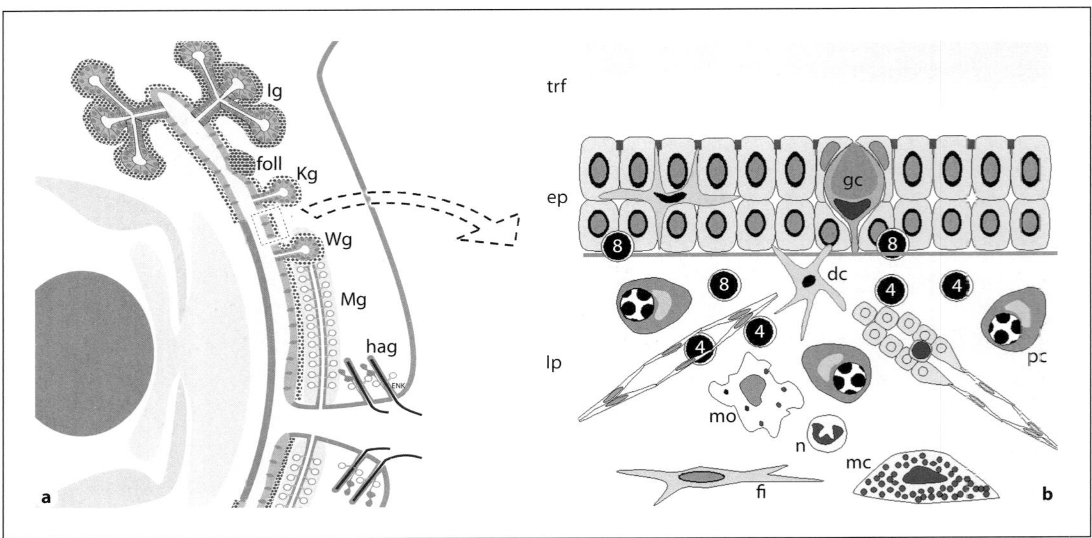

Fig. 1. Topography of eye-associated lymphoid tissue (EALT) at the human ocular surface. **a** EALT extends all along the mucosal surface of the conjunctiva into the periacinar tissue of the lacrimal gland (lg) and the conjunctival accessory lacrimal glands of Krause (Kg) and Wolfring (Wg). Organized accumulations of lymphocytes into lymphoid follicles (foll) also occur. Mg = Meibomian gland; hag = hair associated glands. **b** Diffuse lymphoid tissue can be seen in the lamina propria (lp) and epithelium (ep). Single interspersed lymphocytes and dendritic cells also occur inside the epithelium. In the lamina propria, there are lymphocytes of different subtypes (CD4 and CD8) and plasma cells (pc) together with accessory leukocyte populations, such as macrophages (mo), mast cells (mc), occasional neutrophilic granulocytes (n) and stromal cells (fibroblasts; fi). The lamina propria has vessels of a different kind, and the epithelium is covered by the tear film (trf). gc = goblet cell.

Eye-Associated Lymphoid Tissue (EALT): The Physiological Mucosal Immune System of the Ocular Surface

Ocular Surface

The mucosa of the ocular surface proper (conjunctiva and cornea) is anatomically continuous with its mucosal adnexa, i.e. with the lacrimal and accessory lacrimal glands through the excretory ducts and with the lacrimal drainage system through the lacrimal canaliculi [1]. Together, all 3 organs unite the source of the tears [2] upstream of the conjunctiva, their presumed main target at the ocular surface proper, and their eventual drainage downstream [3] (fig. 1). Hence, this extended ocular surface forms a unit with several functions [for reviews, see 1, 4, 5], e.g. wetting [6], nutrition, cell differentiation and also mucosal immune protection (and its potential deregulation) as considered here.

Dry eye disease represents a widespread disease condition [7–9] that was long misunderstood as an ocular variant of feeling unwell, but which can have a serious

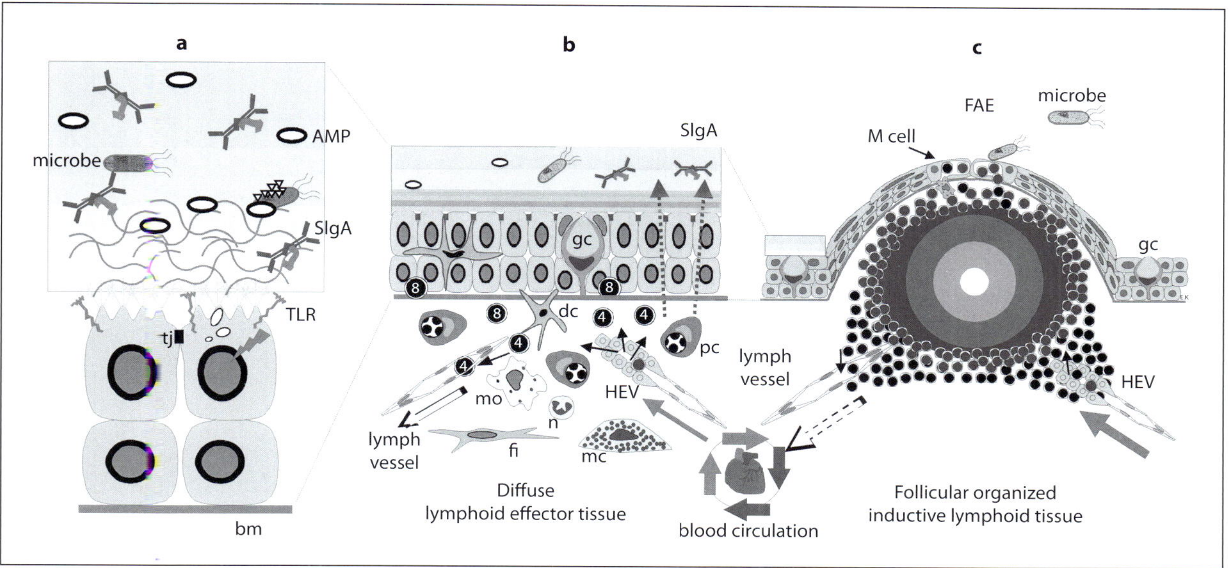

Fig. 2. Arrangement of human conjunctiva-associated lymphoid tissue (CALT). **a** The conjunctiva has several defense systems composed of the integrity of the surface epithelium with the mucin layer, which is enforced by adhering protective molecules (e.g. antimicrobial peptides, AMP) and specific secretory IgA within the tissue and the overlying tear film. SIgA = secretory IgA; TLR = Toll like receptors; bm = basement membrane. **b** CALT consists of a diffuse lymphoid layer composed of mainly effector lymphocytes and also innate effector cells, such as macrophages, mast cells, granulocytes and dendritic cells. This system is supplemented by the lymphoid cells of the specific adaptive immune system, which consists of intraepithelial lymphocytes and lamina propria lymphocytes, such as T cells of different subtypes (CD4+ helper and CD8+ suppressor/cytotoxic cells) and of differentiated B cells (plasma cells) that mainly produce secretory IgA. pc = Plasma cells; dc = dendritic cells; HEV = high endothelial venules; mc = mast cells; gc = goblet cells. **c** Lymphoid follicles and their associated T cell regions, provided with HEV, generate these effector cells. Lymphocytes enter lymphatic tissues preferably via HEV in a regulated fashion and leave via lymphatic vessels, from which they eventually reenter the blood circulation ('recirculation'). Antigen uptake is maintained via a specialized follicle-associated epithelium with antigen-transporting M cells in order to allow ports of regulated antigen entry through the otherwise sealed epithelial surface for the information of the mucosal immune system about the luminal antigen status. Reprinted with permission from Knop E and Knop N, *Encyclopedia of the Eye*, Elsevier, 2010.

impact on ocular surface integrity and may include serious inflammatory reactions [10–12]. In the future, this disease will receive increasing attention in societies where the proportion of the elderly population is growing.

Cell Types in Mucosal Lymphoid Tissue

Mucosa-associated lymphoid tissue (MALT) consists of two sheets: the epithelium and the underlying loose connective tissue of the lamina propria (fig. 2). The epithelium is sealed by apical tight junctions to prevent the entry of foreign materials, including antigens, and constitutes a mechanical barrier that is further enforced by the adhesive properties of a superficial mucin layer [14] and associated antimicrobial peptides and proteins. Hence, impairments in epithelial integrity are a major reason for alterations in mucosal immunity in general, and are also observed in dry eye disease. The epithelium contains leukocytic cells, such as dendritic cells (for antigen-uptake and subsequent presentation) as well as effector T cells, that are mainly located in the basal epithelial layer and are termed, intraepithelial lymphocytes [15].

The lamina propria constitutes a lose collagen meshwork into which the majority of the mucosal leukocytes are embedded (fig. 2b). Stromal fibrocytes produce the collagen fibers and serve for the physical maintenance. In addition, there are bone-marrow-derived cells that have migrated into the tissue from the blood stream [16]. These consist of different cell types, such as lymphocytes of various subtypes (including plasma cells), which are termed 'lamina propria lymphocytes'. In addition, there are accessory leukocytes, such as dendritic cells, macrophages (for phagocytosis of antigens and antigen-presentation), mast cells (that have a role in host defense [17], but are better known for their stimulating action in allergic reactions [18]) and occasional neutrophilic granulocytes. From a wider perspective, the overlying epithelial cells communicate with the leukocytes and have a role in immune reactions [19]. In addition, a large number of macromolecules are present, which are either derived from the bloodstream for nutrition and cell metabolism or produced by the local cells and assist in cell communication (e.g. cytokines and chemokines) [20–22] and protection (e.g. immunoglobulins and antibacterial peptides (AMP)) [23, 24]. Their production is regulated by receptors on the epithelial cells, such as Toll-like receptors (TLR) [25] (fig. 2a).

Arrangement and Function of Mucosal Lymphoid Tissue

The lymphoid cells together with the accessory cells form so-called mucosa-associated lymphoid tissue (MALT), of which two types can be differentiated [15] (fig. 2). The main extension of the mucosal surface is provided with lymphocytes that are diffusely interspersed into the tissue and hence constitute a so-called 'diffuse lymphoid tissue'. T lymphocytes that have differentiated into CD8+ suppressor/cytotoxic cells directly act against antigens, whereas CD4+ T-helper (Th) cells regulate immune response [26]. B cells differentiate into immunoglobulin-producing plasma cells and act indirectly via secreted immunoglobulins, mainly mucosal IgA. Diffuse MALT is mainly populated by differentiated effector cells that can act against antigens; it is therefore termed the 'efferent' arm of mucosal immunity [15] (fig. 2b).

As opposed to the diffuse lymphoid tissue, lymphocytes also form accumulations that are organized into specific functional domains, and are hence termed 'organized lymphoid tissue'. Organized MALT consists of lymphoid follicles composed of mainly B lymphocytes and has parafollicular T cell zones. In organized MALT, naïve lymphocytes that are mature but have not been in contact with antigens are primed by the process of antigen presentation via professional antigen-presenting cells (APC; dendritic cells, macrophages, B cells) and differentiate into effector cells that can act against antigens in different ways. In the follicles, B cells differentiate into antibody-secreting plasma cell precursors, whereas in the parafollicular regions T cells differentiate into the various T cell subtypes. At follicular sites, antigens are taken up from the environment by a specialized follicle-associated epithelium that covers the follicles towards the luminal surface, and hence organized MALT represents the 'afferent' inductive arm of mucosal immunity in a functional sense (fig. 2c), although antigens can also be taken up and later presented by the APC in the diffuse lymphoid tissue.

Differentiated B cells and T cells can act locally inside the tissue but are also eventually distributed (after emigration through lymphatic vessels) throughout the body via the blood stream, and can migrate into the same or other lymphoid organs. This process is known as 'recirculation', and it allows the population of ocular lymphoid tissues with naïve lymphocytes and the exchange of effector cells among different lymphoid organs [27].

Lymphoid Cells at the Human Ocular Surface and Mucosal Adnexa Constitute Eye-Associated Lymphoid Tissue (EALT)

The presence of lymphoid cells as a normal physiological finding in the tissues of the human ocular surface and mucosal adnexa had been under debate until recently, even though they had been mentioned for a long time [28, 29]. This was mainly due to scant knowledge of the mucosal immune system making their functional significance unclear. Understanding was further complicated by the historic misconception that lymphoid cells were, together with the other leukocytes, simply considered as 'inflammatory cells' even though they were observed in every normal tissue [30] and accepted as a normal component, e.g. in the lacrimal and accessory lacrimal glands that are in continuity with the conjunctiva [31, 32].

Later similar relations of lymphoid cell types as in other mucosal organs with a diffuse MALT were found in immunohistological studies of human conjunctiva biopsies [33–35], including the regular presence of mucosa-specific lymphocytes [34, 35]. However, there were different and partly conflicting reports concerning the presence of cell types and the amount location of lymphoid cells, which were most likely based on problems resulting from the minute size of biopsies used and from difficulty in determining their exact location. Also, data from animal tissues was transferred to the human situation [36].

This was only resolved when it was shown in studies on human whole-mount tissues that conjunctiva-associated lymphoid tissue (CALT) [37, 38] and lacrimal drainage-associated lymphoid tissue (LDALT) [3, 39–41] exist, similar to other mucosal organs. The ocular mucosal tissues are termed CALT and LDALT according to the international nomenclature of mucosal immunology [16].

CALT and LDALT form, together with the gland-associated lymphoid tissue of the lacrimal gland, the eye-associated lymphoid tissue (EALT) [1, 3, 4, 42] as a functional unit for ocular surface immune protection and as a new component of the mucosal immune system in the body. This is in line with (for example) gut-associated lymphoid tissue of the intestine or bronchus-associated lymphoid tissue in the airways. Several studies have meanwhile convinced the scientific community that lymphoid cells are a normal and noninflammatory component of the ocular surface [for a review, see 4]. Therefore, lymphoid cells are: (1) resident at the normal human ocular surface; (2) physiologically noninflammatory; (3) continuously involved in the maintenance of protective mucosal immune regulation; (4) do not need acute immigration in order to interact in local immunological processes [1]. These are important differences in contrast to the previous perception that lymphoid cells migrate as 'inflammatory cells' into a primarily lymphocyte-free ocular surface as a secondary or tertiary event in inflammatory disease processes.

EALT Unites the Ocular Surface and Its Mucosal Adnexa

The parts of EALT are connected on different levels (fig. 3): (1) The diffuse lymphoid tissue is physically continuous from the lacrimal gland and accessory lacrimal glands along the conjunctiva into the lacrimal drainage system. (2) The whole ocular mucosal surface shares the same luminal fluid, represented by the tears, and hence shares the same soluble protective factors but conceivably also the same pathogenic repertoire. The latter applies at least to CALT and LDALT due to the fact that the majority of ocular pathogens enter through the open palpebral fissure and float downstream. This may not equally apply to the lacrimal gland because the upstream travel of ocular surface pathogens is conceivably prevented by the tear flow, and this may explain why lymphoid follicles for antigen uptake and effector cell generation are not normally found in the lacrimal gland. (3) The ocular mucosal tissues are also connected by the regulated migration of lymphoid cells ('recirculation') via the numerous small vessels including specialized high endothelial venules [43, 44] that have specific adhesion molecules on the surface of the vascular endothelial cells [45].

Analysis of the topographical distribution of EALT in the conjunctiva shows that it matches the position of the cornea [46] and is in direct contact with the corneal surface when the eye is closed, at night and during blinking. This topography, the fact that the cornea does not contain its own lymphoid cells, and the fact that with the eyes closed during the night corneal integrity is protected by a massive influx of leukocytes and their secretory products [17] strongly suggest that EALT has an important role in the protection of the corneal integrity and health [4].

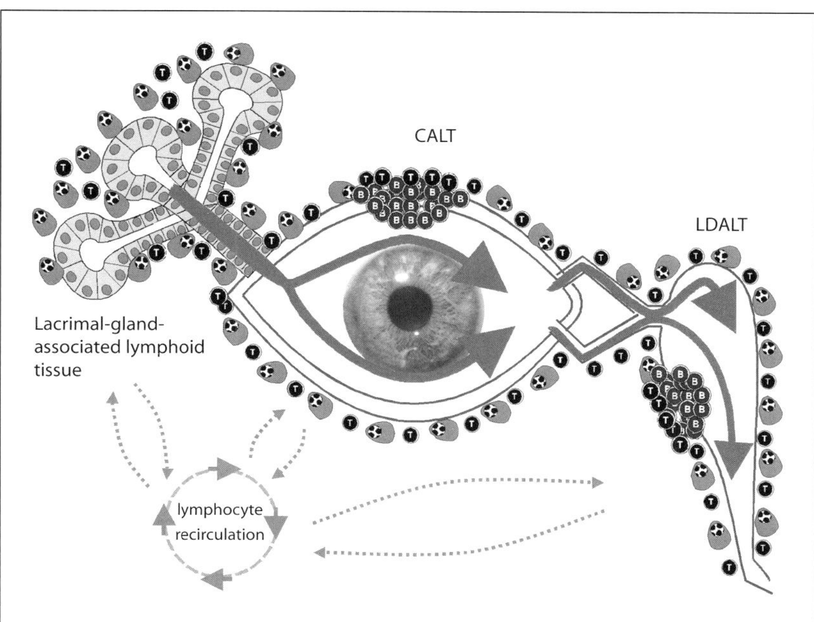

Fig. 3. Eye-associated lymphoid tissue (EALT) consists of CALT at the ocular surface proper and is continuous with the lacrimal and accessory lacrimal glands through their excretory ducts (upstream). Downstream it continues via the lacrimal canaliculi along the lacrimal drainage route as LDALT. A diffuse lymphoid tissue of T lymphocytes (dark round cells) and interspersed IgA-secreting plasma cells (including accessory leukocyte populations; not indicated) occurs along the whole mucosa, whereas lymphoid follicles are physiologically only found in CALT and LDALT. The diffuse lymphoid tissue in EALT is physically continuous and the organs of EALT are also connected via the flow of tears (large arrows) by which they share protective factors as well as pathogens. The organs are furthermore connected by lymphocyte recirculation via specialized vessels (dotted arrows at the bottom; compare with figure 2) with each other and with the other organs of the immune system. Reprinted with permission from Knop E and Knop N, *Immune Response and the Eye*, Karger, 2007.

The main function of ocular surface lymphocytes is (in contrast to previous assumptions) not to generate inflammation, but rather the reverse, i.e. to protect the ocular surface against inflammatory processes that could lead to tissue destruction. Therefore, the ocular mucosal immune system maintains the delicate balance between the tolerance to ubiquitous nonpathogenic antigens and adverse immune reactions against pathogenic microorganisms that involve inflammation and hence endanger ocular surface integrity (fig. 4).

Different Subtypes of Lymphocytes Occur in EALT

Conjunctival lymphocytes in the diffuse lymphoid tissue are mainly CD3+ T cells, whereas most of the CD20+ B cells are restricted to the solitary lymphoid follicles [47].

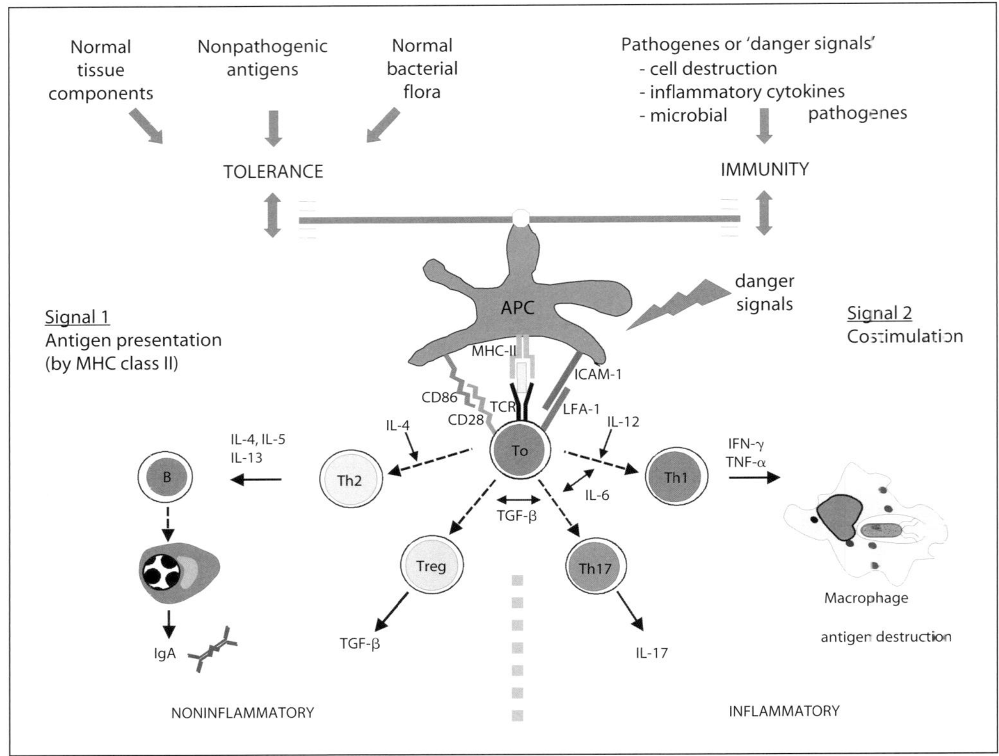

Fig. 4. Ocular surface immune regulation. Immune tolerance to host tissue constituents, nonpathogenic antigens and physiological commensal bacterial flora is essential for tissue integrity in order to avoid unnecessary destructive immune reactions. This must however be in equilibrium with the detection of and defense against pathogens. The fine equilibrium between these 2 important functions is critical for mucosal immunity and the balance is maintained by the mode of antigen-presentation exerted by APC via MHC-class II to naïve (To) lymphocytes that results in the generation of different subtypes of Th cells which produce characteristic cytokine patterns of interleukins (IL). The presentation of an antigen (signal 1) in the context of danger signals as represented by cell destruction, inflammatory cytokines or microbial pathogens leads to the expression of costimulatory molecules (signal 2) and results in inflammatory immune responses by e.g. Th1 or Th17 cells. Regulatory T cells (Treg) suppress inflammatory responses and the normal mucosal noninflammatory IgA response is produced by the differentiation of B cells into plasma cells inside the lymphoid follicles.

They are activated (CD45Ro+, CD25+) [35], and express the human mucosa lymphocyte antigen (HML-1, CD103, integrin αEβ7) [34]. CD8+ cytotoxic/effector lymphocytes are prevalent in the epithelium, and have been proposed to act in a suppressor mode [33] that provides a component of the immune tolerance at the ocular surface. In contrast to the intraepithelial lymphocytes, the lamina propria lymphocytes (fig. 2b) consist predominantly of CD4+ Th cells [34, 35]. Plasma cells account for about one fifth of the conjunctival leukocytes [30], but in absolute numbers they are quite substantial and equivalent to two thirds of those in the lacrimal gland (which had been regarded as the sole source of tear film secretory IgA; SIgA). Therefore, the conjunctiva is able to contribute considerably to its own defense [23] and is not dependent on a passive supply of IgA from the lacrimal gland. Since the number of normal conjunctival lymphocytes is at least three times that of the plasma cells [30], as shown in histology, the number of T cells is therefore considerable (as also verified in immunohistochemistry) [34, 35].

Subtypes and Functions of Conjunctival Lymphocytes Are Determined by the Mode of Antigen Presentation

The generation and modulation of the mucosal immune response is regulated through the process of antigen presentation [48] by APC. These are mainly dendritic cells [49], including Langerhans cells, but also macrophages and B cells. APC present antigens via their MHC class II receptor (MHC-II) to the T cell receptor on naïve T cells. Apart from this signal (signal 1), accessory signals (co-stimulation, signal 2) [50] such as e.g. CD86 or intercellular adhesion molecule 1 (ICAM-1) are also necessary to mount an efficient T cell response. Pathogenic molecular danger signals in the tissue environment – such as molecules from destroyed cells, inflammatory cytokines (e.g. IL-6, TNF-α, INF-γ) or bacterial molecules (e.g. lipopolysaccharide) signal the presence of a nonphysiological and hence dangerous environment to the immune cells and lead to the initiation of an inflammatory immune response. If inflammatory cytokines and other 'danger signals' [50] occur in the tissue, they can bind to (for example) Toll-like receptors and mediate (via intracellular signaling pathways, e.g. NF-kB or protein kinases [51]) the secretion of inflammatory cytokines that skew EALT towards an inflammatory immune response.

Host tissue antigens (self-antigens) are constitutively taken up and presented by APC that are in an immature state, which leads to anergy or deletion of a respective cognate T cell. T cells that detect self-antigens are mainly destroyed in the process of central tolerance inside the primary lymphoid organ (thymus). Since not all antigens of the body are available in the thymus, some autoreactive T cells escape deletion and must be silenced inside the peripheral mucosal organs (peripheral tolerance) in order to avoid autoimmune reactions [52]. Since the presence of danger signals leads to the maturation of dendritic cells with the upregulation of costimulatory molecules on their surface, independent of the nature of the antigen presented on their MHC class II, the presence of chronic inflammation increases the risk that the presentation of autoantigens may lead to the activation (priming) of potential autoreactive T cells. The mode of antigen presentation by APC decides about the subtypes of lymphocytes that are generated from naïve T cells in the priming process (fig. 4).

An important function of mucosal immune regulation is the generation of plasma cells that produce the noninflammatory IgA, which is achieved when antigen presentation occurs under the influence of cytokines, such as IL-4, and results in type 2 Th cells. These interact with B cells and produce cytokines (e.g. IL-4, IL-5, IL-13) that promote the isotype class switch to IgA and the differentiation into IgA-secreting plasma cell precursors [53]. Regulatory T cells (Treg) are generated under the influence of the anti-inflammatory cytokine TGF-β and in turn produce further TGF-β which, together with IL-10, generates a tolerogenic milieu within EALT and prevents inflammation [54, 55]. Interestingly, if the inflammatory cytokine IL-6 is present in addition to TGF-β, this leads – through a switch in signaling pathways – to the preferred generation of inflammatory Th17 cells [56]. These produce the inflammatory IL-17 and other cytokines that are capable of inducing a heavy inflammatory burst against extracellular antigens. Hence, IL-6 appears to be a crucial factor in mucosal immune regulation. If only IL-6 is present, the well-known inflammatory Th1 cells are formed, and these produce inflammatory cytokines [57] (such as IFN-γ and TNF-α) which have the physiological function to activate cells, in particular phagocytes, to destroy intracellular pathogens.

Immune-Mediated Ocular Surface Inflammation Is a Key Event in Advanced Dry Eye Disease

Deregulation of EALT

Epithelial alteration and cell activation due to various stress factors is a central component of dry eye disease, and is certainly well known to every clinician. Intense investigations over recent years have revealed a large body of information on the underlying factors and pathways that link epithelial alteration to inflammatory processes and immune-mediated inflammation.

Various stress mechanisms [51] – e.g. mechanical alteration by increased sheer forces due to tear film defects [58], hyperosmolar stress [59] or exposure to inflammatory cytokines [60] – can activate the ocular surface epithelium. The epithelial cells interpret these events as a threat to tissue integrity, and hence launch mechanisms for immune defense and tissue repair in order to cure this threat. Therefore, they respond by secreting inflammatory cytokines in order to alarm the mucosal immune system, upregulate surface markers (such as MHC-II and ICAM-1 [61]) in order to allow presentation of pathological antigens, and activate proteases (such as matrix-metalloproteinase [60]) in order to digest cell debris and to provide space for the necessarily increased amounts of leukocytes (which is later followed by the onset of repair mechanisms).

If these basically protective mechanisms are constantly overexpressed through continuous stimulation (e.g. by chronic mechanical irritation) as occurs in dry eye disease, this results in a number of unfortunate consequences. The natural tolerogenic bias can be lost and the mucosal immune system becomes deregulated. This conceivably represents the underlying reason for the observed self-perpetuating inflammatory process at the ocular surface and its associated glands [62–64]. This promotes an inflammatory process in which epithelial cells, via MHC-II on their surface, acquire the potential for presentation of antigens, including self-antigens, to

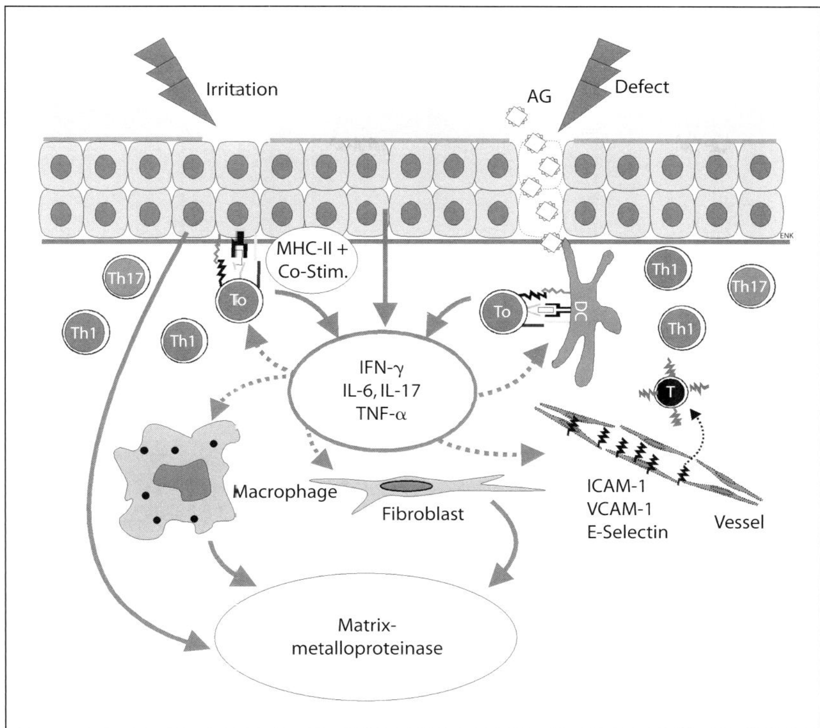

Fig. 5. Deregulation of EALT in ocular surface inflammation. Persistent irritation of the ocular surface epithelium can lead to events that result in a deregulation of EALT. A starting point is (e.g.) tear film deficiency, as found in dry eye disease, that leads to epithelial wounding with eventual activation of the epithelial cells. These respond by secretion of inflammatory cytokines and by expression of the antigen-presenting molecule MHC-II, and they can hence present antigens (including self-antigens) to the resident conjunctival T cells in an inflammatory context. Epithelial defects that breach the physical barrier can lead to the entry of pathogens and nonpathogenic antigens into the tissue, and their subsequent presentation by dendritic cells (DC), also in an inflammatory context, as observed in ocular allergy for example. This contributes to the further accumulation of inflammatory cytokines in the tissue, which is a crucial factor in inflammatory ocular surface disease, and to the generation of inflammatory, potentially autoreactive, types of T cells. Downstream effects are the activation of blood vessel endothelial cells that upregulate adhesion molecules with subsequent recruitment of further leukocytes from the vascular compartment and the activation of bystander cells including stromal cells (fibroblasts and macrophages). These contribute to the activation of matrix metalloproteinases that lead to tissue degradation. All together this constitutes an immune-mediated conjunctival mucosal inflammatory process that is based on deregulation of the physiologically protective EALT. Reprinted with permission from Knop E and Knop N, *The Ocular Surface*, 2005.

resident conjunctival T cells (fig. 5), that may lead to a loss of natural ocular surface immune tolerance [1, 12, 64]. In fact, in experimental inflammatory ocular surface disease, autoreactive T cells are generated that are specific to ocular surface tissue [65] and respective regulatory T cells can prevent the tissue destruction [55].

Increased levels of inflammatory cytokines are associated with further unfortunate consequences, such as: (1) the upregulation of adhesion molecules (like ICAM-1, VCAM-1 or E-selectin) on vascular endothelial cells [61] that results in the recruitment of leucocytes, including further lymphocytes which contribute to the disease [66], from the vascular compartment into the ocular tissues (fig. 5); (2) the increased proliferation of epithelial cells that remain in an immature state and hence lead to the development of squamous metaplasia [67] (fig. 6); (3) impairment of the afferent sensory neural signaling from the ocular surface that results, via a blockade of the lacrimal functional unit [68], in decreased tear production by the lacrimal gland [69].

All together, these events represent an immune-mediated inflammatory episode, orchestrated by deregulation of the resident lymphoid cells of EALT. This is an important common factor in the advanced stages of ocular surface inflammation, including dry eye disease, and can lead to several vicious circles (fig. 6) that propagate the disease [1, 4, 11, 64, 70]. This inflammation is at first subclinical, but tends to amplify if it is not limited in the early stages.

Important starting points for tear film deficiency and consequent ocular surface alteration are a primary deficiency of tear production by the lacrimal gland, which is relatively rare, or a deficiency in the lipid phase of the tear film, which results in increased evaporation of the aqueous tears and hence in an evaporative dry eye (fig. 6). Evaporative dry eye appears more frequently, since a lipid deficiency is reported in about 75% of dry eye patients [71] and in 65% of these it is caused by obstructive meibomian gland dysfunction (MGD) [72]. MGD is mainly based on an obstructive process [73, 74] of the excretory duct and orifice of the meibomian glands [75] that secrete their oils onto the posterior lid margin (see another contribution to this volume) from which they glide onto the tear film as the most superficial phase and limit evaporation [76, 77]. MGD often occurs with minor symptoms and represents an underdiagnosed and underestimated reason for dry eye disease [78, 79]. As judged from its epidemiology and pathophysiology [80], obstructive MGD appears as an important factor for the onset of dry eye (fig. 6) because it: (1) induces epithelial alterations via a hyperevaporative tear deficiency; (2) simultaneously results in hyperosmolarity of the tears, which represents a stress to the ocular surface epithelium, and hence directly activates the epithelial cells to produce inflammatory cytokines [59]; (3) leads to decreased tear clearance and hence an increase in the concentration of inflammatory cytokines in the remaining tears [81] with the results explained above. It can be assumed that an impairment in neural innervation may also apply to the meibomian glands since they share important similarities with the innervation pattern of the lacrimal gland [75]. Therefore, immunomodulated inflammatory processes with all the downstream results may also contribute to the understanding of why the late stages of aqueous deficient and hyperevaporative dry eye share similarities [82].

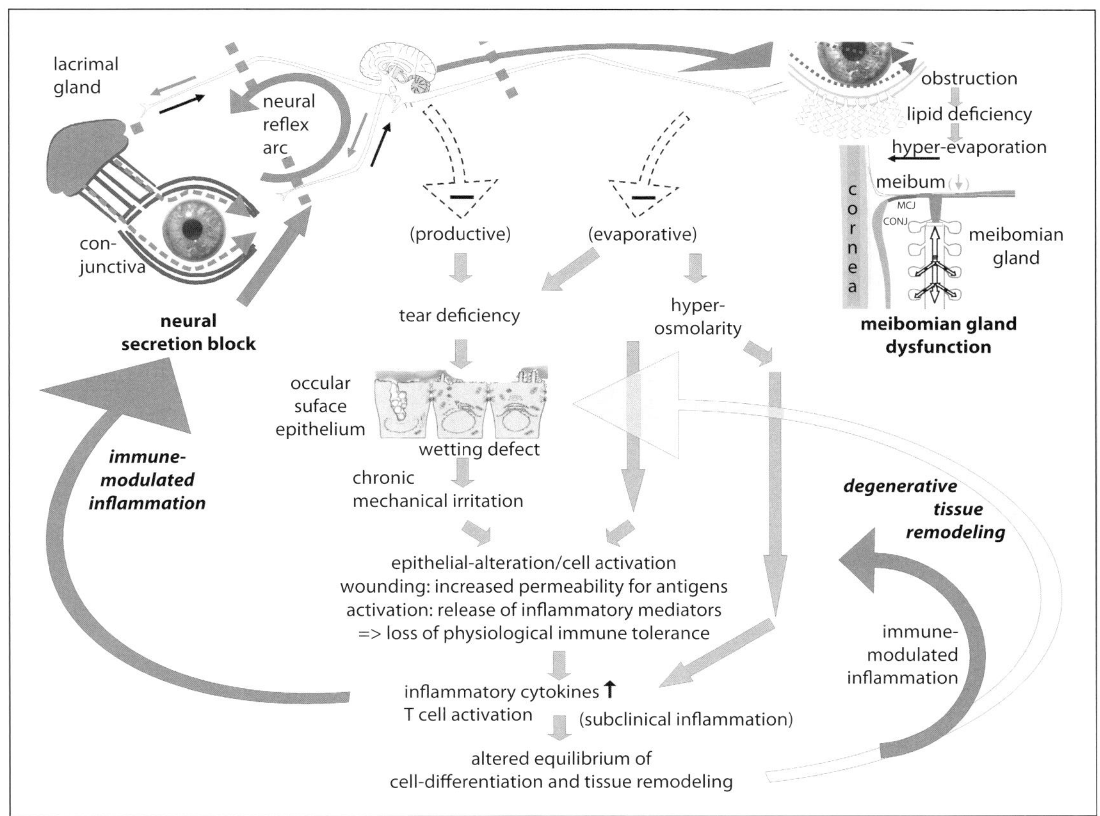

Fig. 6. Vicious circles lead to self-propagation in chronic dry eye disease. The main uniting factor in different forms of ocular surface inflammation, including severe stages of dry eye disease, is the presence of epithelial defects and cell activation with a buildup of inflammatory cytokines and a subclinical inflammation with potential downstream T cell activation and deregulation of the resident mucosal immune system. Different events at the ocular surface can lead to epithelial alterations. These are a secretory or an evaporative tear deficiency that results in chronic mechanical irritation. Evaporative tear deficiency is mainly due to a deficiency in the lipid phase of the tear film due to meibomian gland dysfunction and results, besides a decreased tear volume, in tear hyperosmolarity that directly exerts cell activation and in decreased tear clearance with a buildup of inflammatory cytokines. Persistent subclinical inflammation, modulated by a deregulation of EALT (on the basis of the events explained in figure 5) leads to an altered equilibrium of cell differentiation and tissue remodeling that typically results in squamous metaplasia of the ocular surface. Several vicious circles that originate from these events can negatively reinforce starting points in the sense of vicious circles of immune-modulated inflammation. This aggravates the initial subclinical ocular surface inflammation into an overt form if protective factors are overridden or if this is not limited by timely diagnosis and therapy. An impairment of afferent sensory innervation from the ocular surface due to inflammatory cytokines results in a blockade of the efferent secretory stimuli to the glands and hence aggravates the tear film deficiency. Deterioration of the epithelial differentiation can on the one hand increase the entry of luminal antigens and release host tissue antigens that can be presented in an inflammatory context and hence reinforce immunological deregulation of the mucosal immune system; on the other hand, the lubrication of the surface is negatively influenced.

Physiological Compensatory Mechanisms Can Prevent Disease Progression

The question arises: why do not all patients that have experienced a mild or incipient dry eye condition due to (for example) environmental factors such as low humidity, increased air flow or decreased blinking rate (which frequently occur in ordinary office work at video display terminals in air-conditioned environments) develop severe immune-mediated ocular surface inflammation? The answer is probably quite straightforward, i.e. because in most of us there is a sufficient amount of physiological compensatory factors, such as: (1) the availability of excess tear production capacity in the aqueous, lipid and mucous glands (fig. 1); (2) a sufficient level of androgens that maintain an anti-inflammatory environment at the ocular surface and glands [83] and positively influence the function of the meibomian and other glands [9, 84]; (3) a sufficient regenerative capacity of the tissue; (4) sufficient availability of antigen-neutralizing IgA antibodies by the secretory mucosal immune system [23, 85].

However, if such physiological compensatory factors are reduced (e.g. due to advanced age or hormonal imbalances; in particular, decreased levels of androgen action, increased lid margin degeneration [86] or constant severe environmental desiccating stress [78]), the likeliness of a self-enforcing progressive course of dry eye disease will increase. This may explain why the prevalence of dry eye is generally increased in the aged population, and in particular in females [8].

Acknowledgments

Supported by Deutsche Forschungsgemeinschaft (DFG KN317/11).

References

1 Knop E, Knop N: A functional unit for ocular surface immune defense formed by the lacrimal gland, conjunctiva and lacrimal drainage system. Adv Exp Med Biol 2002;506:835–844.

2 Knop E, Knop N: New techniques in lacrimal gland research: the magic juice and how to drill for it. Opthalmic Res 2008;40:2–4.

3 Knop E, Knop N: Lacrimal drainage associated lymphoid tissue (LDALT): a part of the human mucosal immune system. Invest Ophthalmol Vis Sci 2001; 42:566–574.

4 Knop E, Knop N: The role of eye-associated lymphoid tissue in corneal immune protection. J Anat 2005;206:271–285.

5 Knop E, Knop N: Anatomy and immunology of the ocular surface; in Niederkorn JY, Kaplan HJ (eds): Immune Response and the Eye. Basel, Karger, 2007, pp 36–49.

6 Stern ME, Beuerman RW, Fox RI, Gao J, Mircheff AK, Pflugfelder SC: The pathology of dry eye: the interaction between the ocular surface and lacrimal glands. Cornea 1998;17:584–589.

7 Brewitt H, Sistani F: Dry eye disease: the scale of the problem. Surv Ophthalmol 2001;45(suppl 2):S199-S202.

8 Schaumberg DA, Sullivan DA, Dana MR: Epidemiology of dry eye syndrome. Adv Exp Med Biol 2002; 506:989–998.

9 Sullivan DA: Tearful relationships? Sex, hormones, the lacrimal gland, and aqueous-deficient dry eye. Ocul Surf 2004;2:92–123.

10 Stern ME, Pflugfelder SC. Inflammation in dry eye. Ocul Surf 2004;2:124–130.

11 Knop E, Knop N, Brewitt H: Dry eye disease as a complex dysregulation of the functional anatomy of the ocular surface: new impulses to understanding dry eye disease (in German). Ophthalmologe 2003; 100:917–928.
12 Knop E, Knop N: Influence of the eye-associated lymphoid tissue (EALT) on inflammatory ocular surface disease. Ocul Surf 2005;3:S180–S186.
13 McDermott AM, Perez V, Huang AJ, Pflugfelder SC, Stern ME, Baudouin C, Beuerman RW, Burns AR, Calder VL, Calonge M, Chodosh J, Coster DJ, Dana R, Hazlett LD, Jones DB, Kim SK, Knop E, Li DQ, Mitchell BM, Niederkorn JY, Pearlman E, Wilhelmus KR, Kurie E: Pathways of corneal and ocular surface inflammation: a perspective from the Cullen symposium. Ocul Surf 2005;3:S131–S138.
14 Argueso P, Gipson IK: Epithelial mucins of the ocular surface: structure, biosynthesis and function. Exp Eye Res 2001;73:281–289.
15 Kraehenbuhl JP, Neutra MR: Molecular and cellular basis of immune protection of mucosal surfaces. Physiol Rev 1992;72:853–879.
16 Brandtzaeg P, Pabst R: Let's go mucosal: communication on slippery ground. Trends Immunol 2004; 25:570–577.
17 Sack RA, Beaton A, Sathe S, Morris C, Willcox M, Bogart B: Towards a closed eye model of the preocular tear layer. Prog Retin Eye Res 2000;19:649–668.
18 Stahl JL, Cook EB, Barney NP, Graziano FM: Pathophysiology of ocular allergy: the roles of conjunctival mast cells and epithelial cells. Curr Allergy Asthma Rep 2002;2:332–339.
19 Zhan H, Towler HM, Calder VL: The immunomodulatory role of human conjunctival epithelial cells. Invest Ophthalmol Vis Sci 2003;44:3906–3910.
20 Sack RA, Conradi L, Krumholz D, Beaton A, Sathe S, Morris C: Membrane array characterization of 80 chemokines, cytokines, and growth factors in open- and closed-eye tears: angiotensin and other defense system constituents. Invest Ophthalmol Vis Sci 2005;46:1228–1238.
21 Ono SJ, Nakamura T, Miyazaki D, Ohbayashi M, Dawson M, Toda M: Chemokines: roles in leukocyte development, trafficking, and effector function. J Allergy Clin Immunol 2003;111:1185–1199.
22 Hazlett LD: Pathogenic mechanisms of *P. aeruginosa* keratitis: a review of the role of T cells, Langerhans cells, PMN, and cytokines. DNA Cell Biol 2002;21:383–390.
23 Knop E, Knop N, Claus P: Local production of secretory IgA in the eye-associated lymphoid tissue (EALT) of the normal human ocular surface. Invest Ophthalmol Vis Sci 2008;49:2322–2329.
24 McDermott AM: Defensins and other antimicrobial peptides at the ocular surface. Ocul Surf 2004;2:229–247.
25 Pearlman E, Johnson A, Adhikary G, Sun Y, Chinnery HR, Fox T, Kester M, McMenamin PG: Toll-like receptors at the ocular surface. Ocul Surf 2008; 6:108–116.
26 von Andrian UH, Mackay CR: T-cell function and migration: two sides of the same coin. N Engl J Med 2000;343:1020–1034.
27 Knop E, Knop N: Lymphocyte homing in the mucosal immune system to the eye-associated lymphoid tissue (EALT); in Zierhut M, Sullivan DA, Stern ME (eds): Immunology of the Ocular Surface and Tearfilm. Amsterdam, Swets & Zeitlinger, 2004, pp 35–72.
28 Kessing SV: Mucous gland system of the conjunctiva: a quantitative normal anatomical study. Acta Ophthalmol Copenh 1968;(suppl 95):1–133.
29 Osterlind G: An investigation into the presence of lymphatic tissue in the human conjunctiva, and its biological and clinical importance. Acta Ophthalmol Copenh 1944;23(suppl):1–79.
30 Allansmith MR, Greiner JV, Baird RS: Number of inflammatory cells in the normal conjunctiva. Am J Ophthalmol 1978;86:250–259.
31 Franklin RM, Kenyon KR, Tomasi TB Jr: Immunohistologic studies of human lacrimal gland: localization of immunoglobulins, secretory component and lactoferrin. J Immunol 1973;110:984–992.
32 Wieczorek R, Jakobiec FA, Sacks EH, Knowles DM: The immunoarchitecture of the normal human lacrimal gland: relevancy for understanding pathologic conditions. Ophthalmology 1988;95:100–109.
33 Sacks EH, Wieczorek R, Jakobiec FA, Knowles DM: Lymphocytic subpopulations in the normal human conjunctiva: a monoclonal antibody study. Ophthalmology 1986;93:1276–1283.
34 Dua HS, Gomes JA, Jindal VK, Appa SN, Schwarting R, Eagle RC Jr, Donoso LA, Laibson PR: Mucosa specific lymphocytes in the human conjunctiva, corneoscleral limbus and lacrimal gland. Curr Eye Res 1994;13:87–93.
35 Hingorani M, Metz D, Lightman SL: Characterisation of the normal conjunctival leukocyte population. Exp Eye Res 1997;64:905–912.
36 Chandler JW, Gillette TE: Immunologic defense mechanisms of the ocular surface. Ophthalmology 1983;90:585–591.
37 Knop E, Knop N: MALT tissue of the conjunctiva and nasolacrimal system in the rabbit and human. Vis Res 1996;36:S60.

38 Knop E, Knop N: The mucosa associated lymphoid tissue of the human conjunctiva consists of three components: solitary follicles, crypt associated MALT and a lymphoid layer. Invest Ophthalmol Vis Sci 1997;38:S125.

39 Knop N, Knop E: The lacrimal sac in the rabbit and human is associated with MALT. Vis Res 1996;36: S195.

40 Knop N, Knop E: The MALT tissue of the ocular surface is continued inside the lacrimal sac in the rabbit and human. Invest Ophthalmol Vis Sci 1997; 38:S126.

41 Paulsen FP, Paulsen JI, Thale AB, Schaudig U, Tillmann BN: Organized mucosa-associated lymphoid tissue in human naso-lacrimal ducts. Adv Exp Med Biol 2002;506:873–876.

42 Knop E: Concept of an Eye-Associated Lymphoid Tissue (EALT) as a Functional Unit for Ocular Surface Immune Defence (in German). Hannover, Medical School Hannover, 2001.

43 Knop E, Knop N: Fine structure of high endothelial venules in the human conjunctiva. Ophthalmic Res 1998;30:169.

44 Knop E, Knop N: High endothelial venules are a normal component of lymphoid tissue in the human conjunctiva and lacrimal sac. Invest Ophthalmol Vis Sci 1998;39:S548.

45 Haynes RJ, Tighe PJ, Scott RA, Dua HS: Human conjunctiva contains high endothelial venules that express lymphocyte homing receptors. Exp Eye Res 1999;69:397–403.

46 Knop E, Knop N: Eye-associated lymphoid tissue (EALT) is continuously spread throughout the ocular surface from the lacrimal gland to the lacrimal drainage system (in German). Ophthalmologe 2003; 100:929–942.

47 Knop N, Knop E: Conjunctiva-associated lymphoid tissue in the human eye. Invest Ophthalmol Vis Sci 2000;41:1270–1279.

48 Mougneau E, Hugues S, Glaichenhaus N: Antigen presentation by dendritic cells in vivo. J Exp Med 2002;196:1013–1016.

49 Dana MR: Corneal antigen-presenting cells: diversity, plasticity, and disguise: The Cogan Lecture. Invest Ophthalmol Vis Sci 2004;45:722–727.

50 Matzinger P: The danger model: a renewed sense of self. Science 2002;296:301–305.

51 Pflugfelder SC, De Paiva CS, Tong L, Luo L, Stern ME, Li DQ: Stress-activated protein kinase signaling pathways in dry eye and ocular surface disease. Ocul Surf 2005;3:S154–S157.

52 Steinman RM, Nussenzweig MC: Avoiding horror autotoxicus: the importance of dendritic cells in peripheral T cell tolerance. Proc Natl Acad Sci USA 2002;99:351–358.

53 Brandtzaeg P, Baekkevold ES, Farstad IN, Jahnsen FL, Johansen FE, Nilsen EM, Yamanaka T: Regional specialization in the mucosal immune system: what happens in the microcompartments? Immunol Today 1999;20:141–151.

54 Nesburn AB, Bettahi I, Dasgupta G, Chentoufi AA, Zhang X, You S, Morishige N, Wahlert AJ, Brown DJ, Jester JV, Wechsler SL, BenMohamed L: Functional Foxp3+ CD4+CD25(Bright+) 'natural' regulatory T cells are abundant in rabbit conjunctiva and suppress virus-specific CD4+ and CD8+ effector T Cells during ocular herpes infection. J Virol 2007; 81:7647–7661.

55 Siemasko KF, Gao J, Calder VL, Hanna R, Calonge M, Pflugfelder SC, Niederkorn JY, Stern ME: In vitro expanded CD4+CD25+Foxp3– regulatory T cells maintain a normal phenotype and suppress immune-mediated ocular surface inflammation. Invest Ophthalmol Vis Sci 2008;49:5434–5440.

56 Bettelli E, Oukka M, Kuchroo VK: TH-17 cells in the circle of immunity and autoimmunity. Nat Immunol 2007;8:345–350.

57 Kunert KS, Tisdale AS, Stern ME, Smith JA, Gipson IK: Analysis of topical cyclosporine treatment of patients with dry eye syndrome: effect on conjunctival lymphocytes. Arch Ophthalmol 2000;118:1489–1496.

58 Pflugfelder SC: Tear fluid influence on the ocular surface. Adv Exp Med Biol 1998;438:611–617.

59 Luo L, Li DQ, Corrales RM, Pflugfelder SC: Hyperosmolar saline is a proinflammatory stress on the mouse ocular surface. Eye Contact Lens 2005;31: 186–193.

60 Luo L, Li DQ, Doshi A, Farley W, Corrales RM, Pflugfelder SC: Experimental dry eye stimulates production of inflammatory cytokines and MMP-9 and activates MAPK signaling pathways on the ocular surface. Invest Ophthalmol Vis Sci 2004;45:4293–4301.

61 Gao J, Morgan G, Tieu D, Schwalb TA, Luo JY, Wheeler LA, Stern ME: ICAM-1 expression predisposes ocular tissues to immune-based inflammation in dry eye patients and Sjogrens syndrome-like MRL/lpr mice. Exp Eye Res 2004;78:823–835.

62 Mircheff AK, Wang Y, Jean MS, Ding C, Trousdale MD, Hamm-Alvarez SF, Schechter JE: Mucosal immunity and self-tolerance in the ocular surface system. Ocul Surf 2005;3:182–192.

63 Stern ME, Gao J, Siemasko KF, Beuerman RW, Pflugfelder SC: The role of the lacrimal functional unit in the pathophysiology of dry eye. Exp Eye Res 2004;78:409–416.

64 Knop E, Knop N: Eye associated lymphoid tissue (EALT) and the ocular surface. Proc 5th Int Symp Ocul Pharmacol Ther, Bologna, Medimond, 2004, pp 91–98.

65 Niederkorn JY, Stern ME, Pflugfelder SC, De Paiva CS, Corrales RM, Gao J, Siemasko K: Desiccating stress induces T cell-mediated Sjogren's syndrome-like lacrimal keratoconjunctivitis. J Immunol 2006; 176:3950–3957.

66 Stern ME, Gao J, Schwalb TA, Ngo M, Tieu DD, Chan CC, Reis BL, Whitcup SM, Thompson D, Smith JA: Conjunctival T-cell subpopulations in Sjogren's and non-Sjogren's patients with dry eye. Invest Ophthalmol Vis Sci 2002;43:2609–2614.

67 Pflugfelder SC, Jones D, Ji Z, Afonso A, Monroy D: Altered cytokine balance in the tear fluid and conjunctiva of patients with Sjogren's syndrome keratoconjunctivitis sicca. Curr Eye Res 1999;19:201–211.

68 Stern ME, Beuerman RW, Fox RI, Gao J, Mircheff AK, Pflugfelder SC: A unified theory of the role of the ocular surface in dry eye. Adv Exp Med Biol 1998;438:643–651.

69 Jones DT, Monroy D, Ji Z, Pflugfelder SC: Alterations of ocular surface gene expression in Sjogren's syndrome. Adv Exp Med Biol 1998;438:533–536.

70 Knop E, Knop N, Pleyer U: Clinical Aspects of MALT; in Pleyer U, Mondino B (eds): Uveitis and Immunological Disorders. Berlin, Springer, 2004, pp 67–89.

71 Heiligenhaus A, Koch JM, Kemper D, Kruse FE, Waubke TN: Therapy in tear film deficiencies (in German). Klin Monatsbl Augenheilkd 1994;204:162–168.

72 Shimazaki J, Sakata M, Tsubota K: Ocular surface changes and discomfort in patients with meibomian gland dysfunction. Arch Ophthalmol 1995;113: 1266–1270.

73 Foulks GN, Bron AJ: Meibomian gland dysfunction: a clinical scheme for description, diagnosis, classification, and grading. Ocul Surf 2003;1:107–126.

74 Korb DR, Henriquez AS: Meibomian gland dysfunction and contact lens intolerance. J Am Optom Assoc 1980;51:243–251.

75 Knop N, Knop E: Meibomian glands. I. Anatomy, embryology and histology of the Meibomian glands. Ophthalmologe 2009;106:884–892.

76 Bron AJ, Tiffany JM, Gouveia SM, Yokoi N, Voon LW: Functional aspects of the tear film lipid layer. Exp Eye Res 2004;78:347–360.

77 Knop E, Knop N: Meibomian glands. II. Physiology, characteristics, distribution and function of meibomian oil. Ophthalmologe 2009;106:884–892.

78 Brewitt H, Kaercher T, Rüfer F: Dry eye and blepharitis. Klin Monatsbl Augenheilkd 2008;225: R15–R36.

79 Knop E, Knop N, Brewitt H, Pleyer U, Rieck P, Seitz B, Schirra F: Meibomian glands. III. Meibomian gland dysfunction (MGD) – argument for a discrete disease entity and as an important cause of dry eye. Ophthalmologe 2009;106:966–979.

80 Knop E, Knop N: Meibomian glands. IV. Functional interactions in the pathogenesis of meibomian gland Dysfunction (MGD). Ophthalmologe 2009; 106:980–987.

81 Afonso AA, Sobrin L, Monroy DC, Selzer M, Lokeshwar B, Pflugfelder SC: Tear fluid gelatinase B activity correlates with IL-1alpha concentration and fluorescein clearance in ocular rosacea. Invest Ophthalmol Vis Sci 1999;40:2506–2512.

82 Bron AJ, Yokoi N, Gafney E, Tiffany JM: Predicted phenotypes of dry eye: proposed consequences of its natural history. Ocul Surf 2009;7:78–92.

83 Sullivan DA, Krenzer KL, Sullivan BD, Tolls DB, Toda I, Dana MR: Does androgen insufficiency cause lacrimal gland inflammation and aqueous tear deficiency? Invest Ophthalmol Vis Sci 1999;40:1261–1265.

84 Sullivan DA, Sullivan BD, Evans JE, Schirra F, Yamagami H, Liu M, Richards SM, Suzuki T, Schaumberg DA, Sullivan RM, Dana MR: Androgen deficiency, meibomian gland dysfunction, and evaporative dry eye. Ann N Y Acad Sci 2002;966:211–222.

85 Brandtzaeg P, Baekkevold ES, Morton HC: From B to A the mucosal way. Nat Immunol 2001;2:1093–1094.

86 Hykin PG, Bron AJ: Age-related morphological changes in lid margin and meibomian gland anatomy. Cornea 1992;11:334–342.

87 Barabino S, Shen L, Chen L, Rashid S, Rolando M, Dana MR: The controlled-environment chamber: a new mouse model of dry eye. Invest Ophthalmol Vis Sci 2005;46:2766–2771.

Dr. Nadja Knop
Department of Cell Biology in Anatomy, Hannover Medical School
Carl-Neuberg-Strasse 1
DE–30625 Hannover (Germany)
E-Mail knopnadja@aol.com

Brewitt H (ed): Research Projects in Dry Eye Syndrome.
Dev Ophthalmol. Basel, Karger, 2010, vol 45, pp 40–48

Intravital Multidimensional Real-Time Imaging of the Conjunctival Immune System

U. Gehlser[a,b] · G. Hüttmann[c] · P. Steven[a,b]

[a]Department of Ophthalmology, Campus Lübeck, University Medical Center Schleswig-Holstein, and Institutes of [b]Anatomy and [c]Biomedical Optics, University of Lübeck, Lübeck, Germany

Abstract

The conjunctiva, as a peripheral mucosal surface, is dependent on the migration of immune cells to facilitate an orchestrated immune response. So far, only limited data to visualize these dynamics directly have been obtained, mainly due to technical and experimental restrictions. To investigate migration on a cellular level, the following conditions need to be met: (1) intravital investigations need to be facilitated by suitable microscopic techniques; (2) tissues need to be investigated in three spatial dimensions and over time; (3) data need to contain detailed information about the tissue character. Whereas the use of confocal laser scanning microscopy allows high-resolution imaging of the superficial conjunctival immune system and enables the recording of rapid cellular migration, intravital two-photon microscopy further enables tracking of individual cells and characterization of cells and structures with unique optical features using autofluorescence detection, fluorescence lifetime measurements and second harmonic generation in deep tissue. Based on current results and experimental studies, two-photon microscopy has the potential for general use in basic research and clinical practice, and would greatly enhance possibilities for diagnosing and analyzing inflammatory processes of the ocular surface. In particular, inflammation in common diseases, such as allergy and dry eye, and its progress under treatment could be investigated in detail.

The immune system of the conjunctiva protects the eye from invading pathogens that are constantly present on the ocular surface. In particular, the cellular component of the immune system plays a key role in maintaining a homeostasis between adequate defense in order to fight pathogens and downregulation of the immune response to spare components such as epithelia, goblet cells, etc.

The cellular immune system of the conjunctiva is located within the mucosa as a diffuse and an organized lymphoid tissue. The latter is called 'conjunctiva-associated lymphoid tissue' (CALT), in relation to the term 'mucosa-associated lymphoid tissue' [1]. CALT consists of a lymphoid follicle with B cells, T cells and antigen-presenting cells beneath a lymphoepithelium that is devoid of goblet cells [2]. Using slit-lamp microscopy, CALT follicles can easily be identified as typical mucosal protrusions with a glassy appearance and surrounding capillaries. Longitudinal studies have shown that CALT is not present at birth, but develops during early childhood until almost all young healthy individuals show follicles within their conjunctiva [3–6]. Later in life, the amount of CALT decreases steadily and follicles are only sparsely detected in senility. In contrast to the healthy state, the amount and character of follicles changes dramatically during inflammation of the ocular surface. Conjunctival follicles enlarge and increase in number under specific pathological conditions, such as infections with *Chlamydia*, *Neisseria*, *Bartonella*, *Mycobacteria*, viruses (adeno-associated, pox, herpes, etc.), after challenge with toxic substances, during allergic reactions or in the pathogenesis of dry eye disease [7–9]. A functional role of CALT in the protection of the ocular surface under these conditions is therefore likely, but apart from antigen-uptake studies [for a review, see 10] this has not been addressed in experimental setups so far. It has also been discussed, but not yet proven whether CALT and the ocular surface serve as sites where lymphoid cells (e.g. T or B cells) migrate to from other mucosal areas [11]. In this context, the specificity of IgA in tears was analyzed and found to be directed against bacteria which are not generally found on the ocular surface [12]. These results support the idea that CALT may be part of a common mucosal immune system [13].

An exchange of immune competent cells relies on cellular traffic between different organs or organ compartments. As the conjunctiva represents a peripheral mucosal surface, migration of immune cells to and from the conjunctiva is crucial in facilitating an orchestrated immune response that also includes other parts of the ocular surface, such as the efferent tear ducts and lacrimal gland. Such migration of immune cells is thought to take part in different compartments of the conjunctiva: (1) traffic via blood vessels, especially high-endothelial venules, to the conjunctiva; (2) traffic via lymphoid vessels from the conjunctiva to adjacent lymph nodes; (3) migration of immune cells within diffuse lymphoid tissue and within CALT; (4) migration into intraepithelial pockets of the lymphoepithelium; (5) lymphocytes patrolling the conjunctival epithelium. So far, only limited data has been obtained to visualize these dynamics directly, mainly due to technical and experimental restrictions.

To investigate migration on a cellular level, the following conditions need to be met: (1) investigations have to be conducted on living individuals/animals with the best possible physiological conditions, i.e. intact perfusion, innervation, normal oxygen levels and body temperature; (2) investigations need to be facilitated by suitable microscopic techniques, enabling high-resolution imaging in very deep tissue with no phototoxic side effects; (3) tissues need to be investigated in three spatial dimensions (x, y, z) and over time (t); (4) collected data need to contain detailed information about tissue character (cell subsets, connective tissue components, type of vessels, etc.), e.g. by detection of specific labels or unique tissue features. In the following, intravital high-resolution imaging techniques that are in use in investigations of the ocular-surface-derived immune system are characterized and evaluated according to the criteria described.

In vivo Confocal Laser Scanning Microscopy

Confocal laser scanning microscopy (HRT-adapted Cornea Module, Heidelberg Engineering, Heidelberg, Germany) is a technique that allows minimal invasive imaging of the ocular surface by reflectance of infrared laser light at interfaces of the different tissue structures. Due to the high signal strength, even real-time recording of moving objects in tissues, e.g. intravascular blood flow, is possible. Using this microscope, the conjunctiva of humans has been imaged in health and under pathological conditions, such as allergy, infection or neoplasia [14–18]. Recently, Liang et al. [19] investigated conjunctiva-associated lymphoid tissue in rabbits using in vivo confocal laser scanning microscopy (CLSM). Their interesting study demonstrated an increase in immune cells in CALT following subconjunctival injection of LPS and TNF-α, supporting the theory that CALT plays a key role in ocular surface inflammation. Nevertheless, confocal laser scanning microscopy does not allow the operator to distinguish cell types due to the limited image resolution and the fact that cell-type-related differences in reflectance patterns are too similar to distinguish different cell subsets. Imaging in deeper layers is limited, as scattering based on irregular connective tissue components prevents high-resolution imaging in depths of more than 70–80 μm. Therefore, only lymphoepithelium and superficial parts of the follicle, but not the entire microcompartment of CALT that extends down to 250 μm and further (depending on the species), can be imaged by confocal laser scanning microscopy. Imaging of the cornea, on the other hand, can be taken down to the endothelium, due to the ideal optical properties of this tissue [20, 21]. In summary, the use of CLSM allows high-resolution imaging of the superficial conjunctival immune system and enables the recording of rapid cellular migration, such as intravascular erythrocytes or rolling leucocytes together with an increase in immune cells during inflammation. To analyze different cellular subsets and processes beyond superficial parts of CALT, other imaging techniques that provide more information on the cellular level and at greater tissue depths are necessary. Concerning the conditions mentioned, CLSM meets condition 1 (intravital application), condition 2 in parts (high-resolution, but limited tissue penetration) and condition 3 (image acquisition in 3D: x, y, z) and over time (t). As the image information is based on reflectance only, condition 4 (detection of specific labels or unique features) is not met, although based on the morphology of certain structures (epithelial cells, collagen fibrils, blood vessels, etc.) a certain characterization is feasible. Identification of specific structures or cellular tracking via fluorescent dyes, antibodies or proteins is not possible.

Intravital Two-Photon Microscopy

Another imaging technique for intravital applications was introduced in 1990 by Denk et al. [22]. By using near-infrared femtosecond laser pulses, two-photon microscopy combines the advantages of strong tissue penetration (>250 μm), high resolution (<1 μm) and low phototoxic damage, and is also suitable for intravital investigations in highly scattering tissues. In the past decade, intravital two-photon microscopy was extensively used in animal models to investigate the immune processes in lymph nodes and the spleen. These studies have greatly enhanced our understanding of the dynamics of cell-cell interactions and cellular migration [23–25]. Most experiments were conducted with mice overexpressing fluorescent dyes in particular cell types (e.g. green or yellow fluorescent protein) or following adoptive transfer of fluorescent-labeled cells in order to enable precise differentiation of lymphocytes and dendritic cells, for example. Nevertheless, all other cellular or acellular components that were not labeled with dyes could not be visualized simultaneously.

Intravital Autofluorescence Two-Photon Microscopy

Recently, our group introduced autofluorescence two-photon microscopy to investigate conjunctiva-associated lymphoid tissue of mice without the additional use of fluorescent dyes [26]. This technique is based on the fact that most tissue components contain genuine fluorophores (e.g. NADH, FAD, melanin, etc.). These fluorophores are able to emit autofluorescence following the absorption of near-infrared femtosecond laser pulses used in two-photon microscopy [27]. In addition, collagen can be specifically imaged by second harmonic generation (SHG) of the femtosecond pulses, and lifetime analysis of the excited fluorescence (fluorescence lifetime measurements, FLIM) can be used to further characterize and analyze functional aspects of cells and tissues, e.g. cellular metabolism [28]. By combining autofluorescence two-photon microscopy with SHG and FLIM, we are now able to generate multidimensional data sets of the conjunctival immune system in 3D (x, y, z) and over time (t).

In our setup, we use a commercially available, but modified two-photon microscope (DermaInspect JenLab, Neuengönna, Germany). The DermaInspect consists of a solid-state mode-locked 80-MHz titanium:sapphire laser (MaiTai, Spectra Physics, Darmstadt, Germany) with a tuning range of 710–920 nm. Tissue autofluorescence is usually imaged by exciting the samples at wavelengths between 730 and 826 nm, respectively, and image stacks are recorded with steps of 0.4–1.2 μm. A ×20 objective (IR Achroplan LD 40/0.8 W objective, Carl Zeiss Meditec, Jena, Germany), which is focused by a piezo-driven holder, is used. Larger scale motions of the sample in the x and y directions are performed by computer-controlled stepper motors (Owis,

Staufen, Germany). The autofluorescence is detected by a standard photomultiplier module (H7732, Hamamatsu Photonics, Herrsching, Germany) after passing through a beam splitter (Chroma 640 DCSPXR, AHF Analysentechnik, Tübingen, Germany) and a short-pass filter (BG39, Schott, Mainz, Germany), resulting in a detection bandwidth from 380 to 530 nm. To detect SHG, the excitation is tuned to 826 nm in order to maximize SHG signal strength and transmission of the optics, which are designed for the visible range, and the same photomultiplier with a 413-nm band pass filter (Amko, Tornesch, Germany) is used for suppression of autofluorescence [29].

FLIM is performed by time-correlated single photon counting [30]. Curve fitting with a single exponential decay curve including a deconvolution with the time response of the system (SPCImage 2.6, Becker & Hickl, Berlin, Germany) is used to calculate a mean fluorescence lifetime for each pixel, which is displayed in color-coded images [30]. An animal holder was specially designed to support and orientate experimental animals (mice) in all 3 dimensions (x, y, z). The animal holder is equipped with a heating device to maintain normal body temperature, and additional monitoring of the blood oxygen levels, pulse and breath rate is facilitated by MouseOx (Starr Life Science, Oakmont, Pa., USA). The animals are anesthetized by constantly infusing anesthetics via an intraperitoneal catheter. Assisted ventilation is conducted via tracheotomy and intubation (MiniVent, FMI, Seeheim-Ober Beerbach, Germany).

The secured mouse is placed beneath the two-photon microscope, and the eye is covered with Vidisic Gel (Bausch &Lomb/Dr.Mann Pharma, Berlin, Germany) to bridge the working distance of the water immersion objective used.

Image stacks and time series are recorded and later reconstructed using Imaris Software (Bitplane, Zürich, Switzerland).

3D Reconstruction (x, y, z): Two-photon microscopy enables imaging of entire lymphoid follicles including the lymphoepithelium, follicle and adjacent lymph and blood vessels (fig. 1a) up to a depth of approximately 200 μm in this model. By detecting tissue autofluorescence, epithelial cells can be distinguished from lymphocytes, macrophages and connective tissue components. In contrast to lymphocytes, macrophages demonstrate a strong autofluorescence signal that is based on lysosomes within the cytoplasm (fig. 1b). Virtually empty vessels with a large lumen represent lymphatics, whereas blood vessels are filled with erythrocytes (fig. 1b).

To investigate dynamics of immune cells, time series (x, y, t) are recorded. Within the diffuse lymphoid tissue of the conjunctiva, individual cells migrate preferentially along connective tissue fibers. Investigation of individual lymphocytes within the lymphoepithelium and the follicle show surprisingly high velocities, at a mean of 12 μm/min. In contrast, antigen-presenting cells within CALT do not show any migration, but stay localized in the centre of the follicle. Within intraepithelial pockets, lymphocytes migrate rapidly and demonstrate a rotation-like pattern. The exchange of lymphocytes between epithelial pockets and the subepithelial space or follicle

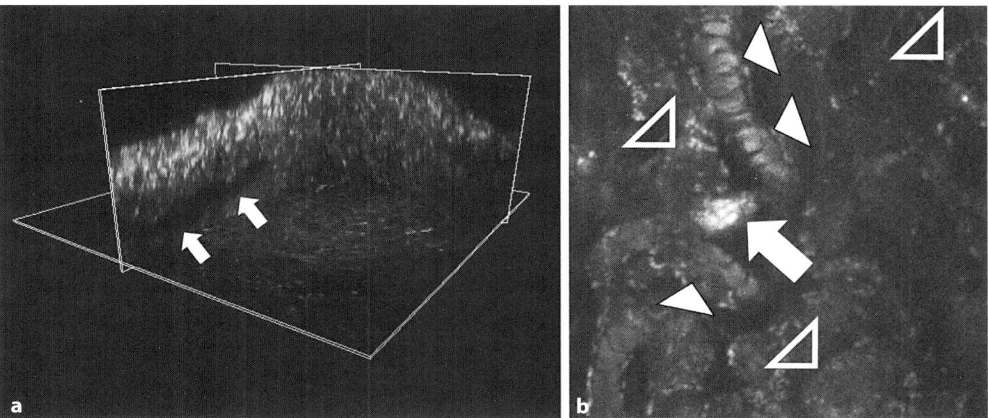

Fig. 1. Two-photon microscopy of CALT. **a** 3D-reconstruction of entire CALT with lymphoepithelium, follicle and adjacent lymphoid vessels (arrows). Edge length: x, y = 380 μm, z = 220 μm. **b** Section through parafollicular zone. Lymphocytes (hollow arrowheads) demonstrate a weak autofluorescence signal in contrast to macrophages (arrow) that contain strong fluorescing lysosomes. Erythrocytes (solid arrowheads) are clearly visible within capillaries.

is currently under investigation. As lymphocytes contain only a few mitochondria within their cytoplasm, the autofluorescence signal that is based on the amount of NADH within the mitochondria is therefore weak. To enhance the contrast between such cells and surrounding tissue components, such as epithelial cells and connective tissue fibers, fluorescent dyes can additionally be introduced in this multidimensional setup. The approach combines the advantages of autofluorescence imaging of the whole microcompartment and the labeling of isolated cells or structures. Intravenous injection of Hoechst dye (33342) results in unspecific nuclear staining of different immune cells. Intravital two-photon microscopy then allows tracking of individual cells with a strongly fluorescing nucleus within (for example) the epithelium of the conjunctiva (fig. 2). These cells show amoeboid migration patterns to move and squeeze their cellular body through narrow gaps between epithelial cells of the basal epithelium.

Apart from using artificial dyes, measurement of FLIM can be used to enable optical fingerprinting of individual cells. The decay times of cellular or acellular components are related to the composition of different fluorophores within the structure of interest. Recently, we were able to show that (for example) goblet cells contain fluorophores with significantly longer fluorescence lifetimes than surrounding epithelial cells. Erythrocytes instead have a extremely short fluorescence lifespan, and macrophages combine distinct lifetime signals in contrast to epithelial cells [31]. FLIM adds valuable information by allowing the operator to distinguish (for example) macrophages, lymphocytes and intravascular erythrocytes by different lifetime spectra. Ongoing studies focus on the identification of specific optical fingerprints in order

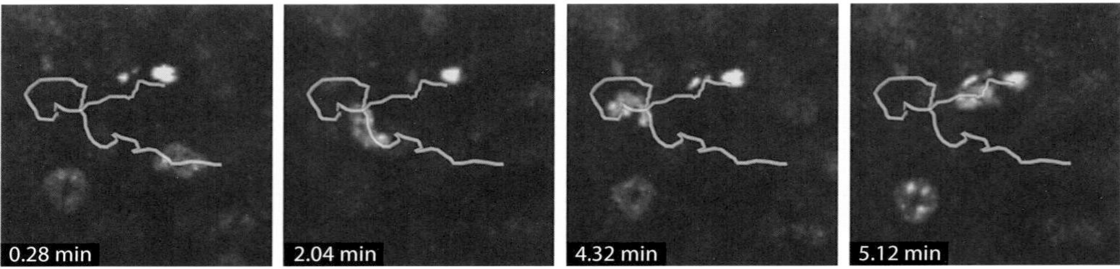

Fig. 2. Intravital two-photon microscopy of the conjunctival epithelium (view perpendicular to the surface). Intraepithelial cells are non-specifically labeled with a fluorescent nuclear stain (Hoechst dye) to enhance the contrast. An individual cell moves through the basal cell layer with an amoeboid migration pattern over a period of approximately 5 min.

to identify and follow cells without the absolute requirement of artificial fluorescent dyes during intravital two-photon microscopy.

In summary, autofluorescence two-photon microscopy combines technical and experimental properties that meet all conditions mentioned earlier: intravital high-resolution imaging at large tissue depths and with low phototoxic damage, image acquisition is facilitated in three spatial dimensions and over time, and tissue features based on autofluorescence, FLIM or SHG, or optional specific labeling with fluorescent dyes. By using two-photon microscopy for intravital investigations, multidimensional image acquisition (x, y, z, t, autofluorescence, FLIM, SHG, fluorescent dyes) allows detailed analysis of tissue characteristics and also dynamics that are of crucial interest in ophthalmological research of the ocular surface.

Future Directions and Implications

Two-photon microscopy detects autofluorescence that is displayed only in gray-scale intensity images. Currently modifications of two-photon microscopes include the additional spectral segregation of the emitted autofluorescence by multi-channel detectors. By doing this, even more information about the investigated tissue is obtained, increasing the opportunity for advanced optical fingerprinting in another dimension (spectral imaging).

At the moment, two-photon microscopy is mainly used in basic immunological research. Based on the promising results, we conclude that besides further experimental projects, use in clinical practice would greatly enhance possibilities for diagnosing and analyzing inflammatory processes of the ocular surface. In particular, inflammation in common diseases, such as allergy and dry eye, and its progress under treatment could be investigated. By identifying suitable excitation wavelengths and detection modes (autofluorescence, +/− FLIM, +/− SHG) and based on a further decrease in costs for single-wavelength femtosecond lasers, a clinical device for multidimensional two-photon microscopy of the ocular surface may be seen in the near future. Hereby, a combination of CLSM and two-photon microscopy would combine the fast scanning properties of the CLSM in localization of (e.g.) CALT with two-photon microscopy for further detailed analysis of the inflammatory cell subsets.

References

1 McDermott MR, Bienenstock J: Evidence for a common mucosal immunologic system. I. Migration of B immunoblasts into intestinal, respiratory, and genital tissues. J Immunol 1979;122:1892–1898.

2 Knop N, Knop E: Conjunctiva-associated lymphoid tissue in the human eye. Invest Ophthalmol Vis Sci 2000;41:1270–1279.

3 Osterlind G: An investigation into the presence of lymphatic tissue in the human conjunctiva, and its biological and clinical importance. Acta Ophthalmol (Copenh) 1944;23:1–79.

4 Wotherspoon AC, Hardman-Lea S, Isaacson PG: Mucosa-associated lymphoid tissue (MALT) in the human conjunctiva. J Pathol 1994;174:33–37.

5 Hingorani M, Metz D, Lightman SL: Characterisation of the normal conjunctival leukocyte population. Exp Eye Res 1997;64:905–912.

6 Dua HS, Gomes JA, Jindal VK, Appa SN, Schwarting R, Eagle RC Jr, Donoso LA, Laibson PR: Mucosa specific lymphocytes in the human conjunctiva, corneoscleral limbus and lacrimal gland. Curr Eye Res 1994;13:87–93.

7 Darrell RW: Follicular conjunctivitis; in Darrell RW (ed): Viral Diseases of the Eye. Philadelphia, Lea & Febiger, 1985, pp 296–311.

8 Krachmer JH, Mannis MJ, Holland EJ: Cornea. Mosby, 2004.

9 Paulsen FP, Schaudig U, Thale AB: Drainage of tears: impact on the ocular surface and lacrimal system. Ocul Surf 2003;1:180–191.

10 Steven P, Gebert A: Conjunctiva-associated lymphoid tissue – current knowledge, animal models and experimental prospects. Ophthalmic Res 2009;42:2–8.

11 Knop E, Knop N: The role of eye-associated lymphoid tissue in corneal immune protection. J Anat 2005;206:271–285.

12 Burns CA, Ebersole JL, Allansmith MR: Immunoglobulin A antibody levels in human tears, saliva, and serum. Infect Immun 1982;36:1019–1022.

13 Chodosh J, Kennedy RC: The conjunctival lymphoid follicle in mucosal immunology. DNA Cell Biol 2002;21:421–433.

14 Malandrini A, Martone G, Traversi C, Caporossi A: In vivo confocal microscopy in a patient with recurrent conjunctival intraepithelial neoplasia. Acta Ophthalmol 2008;86:690–691.

15 Hu Y, Adan ES, Matsumoto Y, Dogru M, Fukagawa K, Takano Y, Tsubota K, Fujishima H: Conjunctival in vivo confocal scanning laser microscopy in patients with atopic keratoconjunctivitis. Mol Vis 2007;13:1379–1389.

16 Messmer EM, Mackert MJ, Zapp DM, Kampik A: In vivo confocal microscopy of normal conjunctiva and conjunctivitis. Cornea 2006;25:781–788.

17 Pichierri P, Martone G, Loffredo A, Traversi C, Polito E: In vivo confocal microscopy in a patient with conjunctival lymphoma. Clin Experiment Ophthalmol 2008;36:67–69.

18 Wakamatsu TH, Sato EA, Matsumoto Y, Ibrahim OM, Dogru M, Kaido M, Ishida R, Tsubota K: Conjunctival in vivo confocal scanning laser microscopy in patients with Sjogren syndrome. Invest Ophthalmol Vis Sci 2010;51:144–150.

19 Liang H, Baudouin C, Dupas B, Brignole-Baudouin F: Live conjunctiva-associated lymphoid tissue analysis in rabbit under inflammatory stimuli using in vivo confocal microscopy. Invest Ophthalmol Vis Sci 2010;51:1008–1015.

20 Stave J, Guthoff R: Imaging the tear film and in vivo cornea: initial results with a modified confocal laser scanning ophthalmoscope (in German). Ophthalmologe 1998;95:104–109.

21 Stave J, Zinser G, Grummer G, Guthoff R: Modified Heidelberg retinal tomograph HRT: initial results of in vivo presentation of corneal structures (in German). Ophthalmologe 2002;99:276–280.

22 Denk W, Strickler JH, Webb WW: Two-photon laser scanning fluorescence microscopy. Science 1990;248:73–76.

23 Mrass P, Weninger W: Immune cell migration as a means to control immune privilege: Lessons from the CNS and tumors. Immunol Rev 2006;213:195–212.

24 Cahalan MD, Parker I, Wei SH, Miller MJ: Two-photon tissue imaging: seeing the immune system in a fresh light. Nat Rev Immunol 2002;2:872–880.
25 Hugues S, Fetler L, Bonifaz L, Helft J, Amblard F, Amigorena S: Distinct T cell dynamics in lymph nodes during the induction of tolerance and immunity. Nat Immunol 2004;5:1235–1242.
26 Steven P, Rupp J, Hüttmann G, Koop N, Lensing C, Laqua H, Gebert A: Experimental induction and three-dimensional two-photon imaging of conjunctiva-associated lymphoid tissue. Invest Ophthalmol Vis Sci 2008;49:1512–1517.
27 Piston DW, Masters BR, Webb WW: Three-dimensionally resolved NAD(P)H cellular metabolic redox imaging of the in situ cornea with two-photon excitation laser scanning microscopy. J Microsc 1995;178:20–27.
28 Skala MC, Riching KM, Gendron-Fitzpatrick A, Eickhoff J, Eliceiri KW, White JG, Ramanujam N: In vivo multiphoton microscopy of NADH and FAD redox states, fluorescence lifetimes, and cellular morphology in precancerous epithelia. Proc Natl Acad Sci USA 2007;104:19494–19499.
29 Morishige N, Petroll WM, Nishida T, Kenney MC, Jester JV: Noninvasive corneal stromal collagen imaging using two-photon-generated second-harmonic signals. J Cataract Refract Surg 2006;32:1784–1791.
30 Becker W: Advanced time-correlated single photon counting techniques. Berlin, Springer, 2005.
31 Steven P, Müller M, Koop N, Rose C, Hüttmann G: Comparison of Cornea Module and DermaInspect for noninvasive imaging of ocular surface pathologies. J Biomed Opt 2009;14:064040.

Dr. Philipp Steven
Department of Ophthalmology, University Medical Center Schleswig-Holstein
Campus Lübeck, Ratzeburger Allee 160
DE–23538 Lübeck (Germany)
Tel. +49 451 500 4015, Fax +49 451 500 4952, E-Mail p.steven@uk-sh.de

Brewitt H (ed): Research Projects in Dry Eye Syndrome.
Dev Ophthalmol. Basel, Karger, 2010, vol 45, pp 49–56

Generation of Two- and Three-Dimensional Lacrimal Gland Constructs

S. Schrader[a,b,d] · L. Liu[c] · K. Kasper[e] · G. Geerling[e]

[a]Cells for Sight Transplantation and Research Programme, Ocular Biology and Therapeutics, UCL Institute of Ophthalmology, and [b]Moorfields Eye Hospital NHS Foundation Trust, London, and [c]Academic Unit of Ophthalmology, Institute of Biomedical Research, College of Medical and Dental Sciences, University of Birmingham, Birmingham, UK; [d]Department of Ophthalmology, University of Lübeck, Lübeck, and [e]Department of Ophthalmology, Julius Maximilian University Würzburg, Würzburg, Germany

Abstract

Aqueous tear deficiency due to lacrimal gland insufficiency is one of the major causes of dry eye. In severe cases, such as Sjoegren's syndrome, Stevens-Johnson syndrome or ocular cicatricial pemphigoid, therapy with artificial tears can be insufficient to relieve severe discomfort. Engineering a lacrimal gland construct may offer a suitable alternative transplant with a tear-like secretion. However, the reconstruction of a complex structure such as the lacrimal gland is challenging, and a lacrimal gland substitute must meet several criteria. It has to contain enough functional lacrimal gland cells to produce an adequate amount of tear fluid, and a suitable matrix is needed to deliver the cells to the patient. The growing field of regenerative medicine offers promising new prospects for lacrimal gland reconstruction. This article summarizes our group's current work in developing models for lacrimal gland reconstruction, and also discusses the perspectives of a tissue-engineered lacrimal gland for future applications.

Dry eye disease, also known as keratoconjunctivitis sicca or more recently dysfunctional tear syndrome, is a multifactorial disease of the tears and ocular surface that results in symptoms of discomfort, visual disturbance and tear film instability with potential damage to the ocular surface. It has a diverse etiology and the major categories are aqueous-deficient and evaporative dry eyes. Lacrimal gland insufficiency is one of the major causes of the former category resulting from primary lacrimal gland dysfunction such as congenital alacrima and familial dysautonomia or secondary causes including lacrimal gland infiltration, ablation and denervation [1]. Common treatment options, such as tear substitutes, punctal plugs or moisture-chamber spectacles, rarely provide sufficient continuous relief in patients with severe lacrimal gland dysfunction. A possible long-term solution for this diverse group of patients might be a bioartificial lacrimal gland microsystem [2]. Like any other engineered tissue, a constructed lacrimal gland requires two main components: differentiated cells able to secrete tears to moisturize the ocular surface and a scaffold to maintain the morphological and physiological properties of the cells. Currently the main cell source for a tissue-engineered lacrimal gland is lacrimal gland acinar cells, and these have been successfully isolated from various species, such as rat, rabbit and human [3–5]. The cell morphology, growth, differentiation and tear secretion largely depend on the cell culture condition and the type of scaffold. A variety of polymeric substrata including collagen I, Matrigel, silicone, copolymers of PLGA (poly-D,L-lactide-co-glycolide; 85:15 and 50:50), PLLA (poly-L-lactic acid) and Thermanox plastic have been compared to determine their capability of supporting growth and morphological development of the lacrimal gland acinar cells. PLLA was found to be favorable compared to other polymers [6]. Amniotic membrane (AM) has been successfully used for ocular surface reconstruction and for treating ocular surface abnormalities, such as persistent epithelial defects, pterygium and symblepharon [7]. It might offer a suitable alternative as a carrier for lacrimal gland acinar cells in vitro as it has been shown to support cell growth and sustain the secretory response to carbachol stimulation for up to 21 days [8].

Tissue engineering is an emerging field in the area of biotechnology that combines the principles and methods of life sciences and has the potential to represent the future of transplantation in medicine. Stem cells, especially embryonic stem cells and pluripotent stem cells, have the potential to be a renewable source for tissue engineering and great progress has been made towards differentiating stem cells to specific cell lineages in recent years [9, 10]. This article summarizes our group's current work in developing models for lacrimal gland reconstruction, and also discusses the possibilities offered by a tissue-engineered lacrimal gland in future applications.

AM-Based Two-Dimensional Lacrimal Gland Model

AM, the innermost layer of the placenta, has successfully been used as an extracellular matrix for cell cultivation. AM consists of three layers: the epithelium, a thick basement membrane and an avascular stroma; several in-vitro studies have shown that AM supports the adhesion, migration, differentiation and proliferation of epithelial cells [11–13]. The AM has been found to be a suitable transplant in various conditions, such as pterygium surgery, ocular surface reconstruction, or treatment of persistent epithelial defects [14–16]. It has also been used as a carrier for transplantation of limbal stem cells, oral mucosal and conjunctival epithelial cells [12, 17, 18]. Our group evaluated the growth pattern and the secretory function of lacrimal gland acinar cells on AM. We were able to show that lacrimal gland acinar cells, when seeded on AM, formed small cell clusters, which increased in

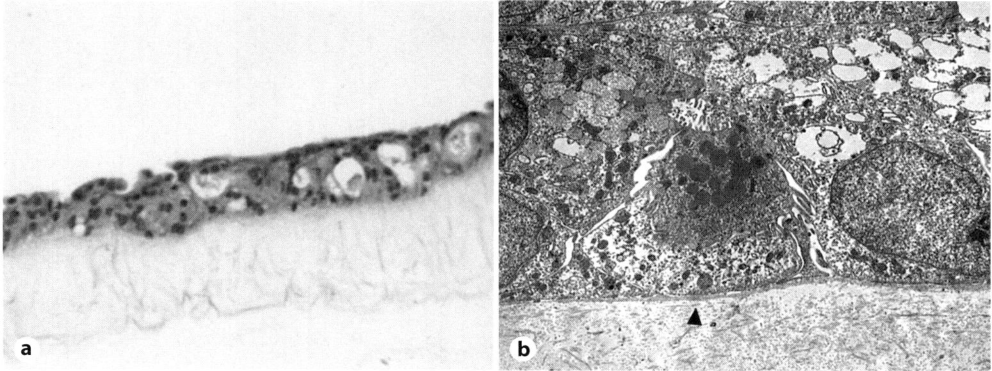

Fig. 1. **a** Acinar cells after 14 days of culture, forming a coating of several cell layers on the AM. ×20. **b** Electron microscopic image after 7 days of culture, showing acinar cells on the basement membrane of the AM (arrowhead) forming a acinus-like structure with a central lumen. The cells show polarity with a basal nucleus, apical secretory granules and microvilli on their apical surfaces. ×3,000.

size and established a coating of several cell layers on parts of the AM (fig. 1a). The cells retained their histotypic features for up to 28 days of culture, but necrotic cells were noted in the centers of the clusters. Electron microscopy revealed cells forming acini-like structures with a central lumen. Cells showed polarity with a basal nucleus, apical secretory granules and microvilli on their apical surfaces (fig. 1b). However, changes in the apical cell layers to small spindle shaped cells were also observed in parts of the AM. These morphological changes seemed to mainly affect the superficial layers, whereas the cells that had contact with the AM predominately retained their acinar cell morphology. Stimulation with carbachol showed a strong ß-hexosaminidase release until day 7, with a decreasing secretory function detectable until day 21 [8].

Three-Dimensional Lacrimal Gland Model

Rotary Cell Culture Systems were originally designed to predict the impact of the microgravity environment in space upon the culture of cells [19]. They have proven to support the development of 3D tissue structures, the formation of cell-cell contacts [20, 21] and to provide an environment of low shear force and high mass transfer of nutrients and metabolic wastes [22]. In our experiments, simulated microgravity promoted the development of spheroidal aggregates with a mean diameter of 384.6 ± 111.8 μm after 7 days (fig. 2a). The spheroids consisted of organized acinar cell conglomerates with fine granulation in their cytoplasm, typical for secreting cells (fig. 2b), and electron microscopy revealed organization

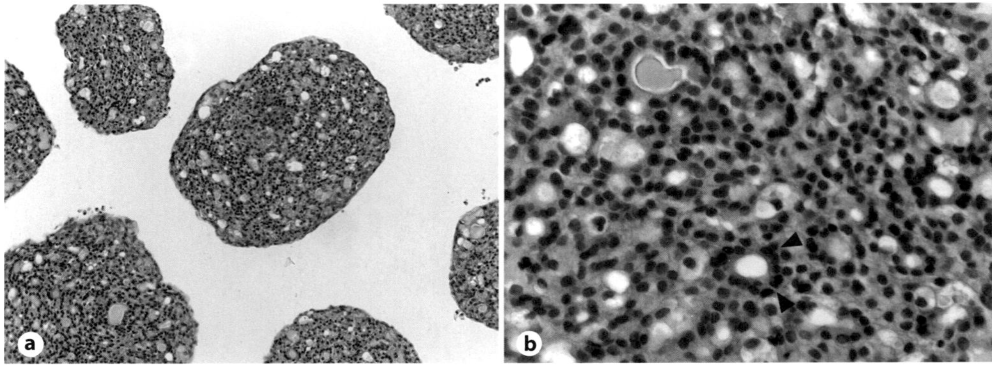

Fig. 2. **a** Spheroidal aggregates containing viable lacrimal gland acinar cells after 14 days of culture. ×10. **b** Organized cell communities with acinus-like structures (arrowheads) inside a spheroid after 14 days of culture. ×40.

into acinus-like structures with a central lumen. However, in the center of the spheroids, an area of apoptosis was noted at all time points. The development of apoptotic centers inside the spheroids correlated with their size. On days 14, 21 and 28, the diameter of the spheroids containing apoptotic centers was significantly higher than in spheroids without apoptotic centers. Also, the duration of the culture period seemed to play a role, as the ratio of apoptosis inside the spheroids increased significantly between days 14 and 21 and between days 21 and 28. The morphological results correlated with the secretory response to stimulation with carbachol, as the secretory response of the cells decreased during the culture period [23].

Colony-Forming Capacity of Lacrimal Gland Cells

Using adult stem cells as a source of tissue regeneration has been proposed for many tissue types, including the ocular surface epithelia [24, 25] and glandular tissues (as the salivary glands and the pancreas have shown that progenitor cells are present in these tissues and involved in their regeneration [26–28]). There is also evidence that the lacrimal gland contains progenitor cells and that these cells are capable of tissue repair after injury [29]. Our group performed colony-forming efficiency assays to evaluate the ability of lacrimal gland acinar cells to form colonies when seeded into 6-well plates and cultured in the presence of a growth-arrested 3T3 feeder layer. Our results showed that large and smooth colonies with a diameter of up to 6.7 mm were formed by the lacrimal gland cells (fig. 3a). Assessment of cytokeratin expression by immunostaining showed strong positivity for pan cytokeratin, confirming the epithelial origin of the cells inside the colonies (fig. 3b).

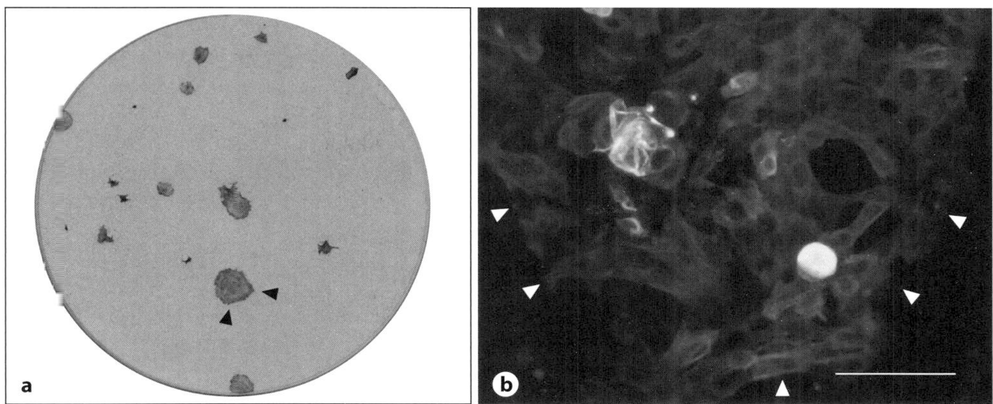

Fig. 3. **a** Colony-forming efficiency assay showing large lacrimal gland acinar cell colonies (arrowheads). **b** Immunostaining of cell colony (arrowheads), showing lacrimal gland cells which are strongly positive for the epithelial cell marker pan cytokeratin (green). Scale bar = 100 µm.

Discussion and Future Prospects

Transplantation of the lacrimal gland is hardly feasible due to the short ischemia time of the tissue of less then 6 h and the small dimension of the gland's vascular supply. In the absence of a suitable lacrimal gland transplant, salivary glands have instead been used to treat patients with otherwise intractable severe dry eye [30]. However, the substantial differences between tears and saliva in their electrolyte and protein composition result in persistent ocular surface disease and can induce a microcystic epithelial edema.

Engineering a lacrimal gland construct may offer a suitable alternative transplant with a tear-like secretion. However, reconstruction of a complex structure such as the lacrimal gland is challenging and a lacrimal gland substitute must meet several criteria. It has to contain enough functional lacrimal gland cells to produce an adequate amount of tear fluid to keep the ocular surface moist, and a suitable matrix is needed to deliver the cells to the patient. Also, a guidance structure may be required to deliver the tear fluid from the construct site to the ocular surface. For long-term success of a tissue-engineered lacrimal gland construct, a progenitor cell population is also likely to be needed to ensure renewal of the lacrimal gland cell population and thus long-term graft functionality. As the maintenance of stem cells relies on a variety of intercellular interactions, the external environment and the underlying mesenchyme together forming particular microenvironments known as 'niches' [31], the matrix also needs to act as an artificial niche environment to preserve the progenitor cell population.

AM meets many criteria of an ideal matrix, as several in vitro studies have shown that AM supports adhesion, migration and proliferation of epithelial cells [11–13].

There is evidence that it may preserve epithelial progenitor cells in vitro [32, 33] and AM-based epithelial cell sheets have already been used for ocular surface reconstruction [17, 18, 24, 34]. According to our experiments, it seems that AM facilitates the formation of 3D cell clusters and stratified epithelium of lacrimal gland acinar cells. This does not exactly replicate the physiology of the intact gland, where the acinar epithelium is single-layered and only becomes stratified in the distal duct segments, and it may influence the secretory activity as presumably the deeper cell layers only have a small impact on the secretion due to the diffusion barrier of the apical cell layers. If such a construct is transplanted directly to the ocular surface, it is also important to know how the lacrimal gland cells would cope with the ocular surface environment where epithelial cells are not only exposed to an air-liquid interface, but also to mechanical stress (such as blinking-induced shear forces). These potential problems will have to be addressed in further studies.

A 3D lacrimal gland construct where the acinar cells are not directly exposed to the ocular surface might mimic the physiological situation more closely, and therefore be more suitable as a lacrimal gland substitute. Work by our group has shown that a Rotary Cell Culture System promotes the development of 3D cell spheroids containing viable acinar cells up to 28 days. Due to the evolving apoptosis inside the spheroids, it is unlikely that such simple 3D cell communities of lacrimal gland acinar cells can serve as tissue equivalents for clinical transplantation, but it shows that a simulated microgravity environment is capable of forming 3D lacrimal gland cell communities of relatively large size, which is essential for a possible lacrimal gland substitute as high cell numbers will probably be needed for sufficient lubrication of the ocular surface. As a variety of cell functions – including proliferation, migration and differentiation – are regulated by cellular interactions with the extracellular matrix, the use of 3D scaffolds as an extracellular matrix may help to retain a differentiated phenotype and cell function in vitro [35]. This may also improve the mass transfer and oxygen supply in the center of the tissue and thus avoid central apoptosis.

The growing field of regenerative medicine offers promising new developments in lacrimal gland reconstruction, and our future work will focus on new matrices for lacrimal gland cell delivery, identification and characterization of lacrimal gland progenitor cells, and optimization of culture conditions to maintain and expand functional lacrimal gland cells in vitro.

References

1 Perry HD: Dry eye disease: pathophysiology, classification, and diagnosis. Am J Manag Care 2008;14:79–87.

2 Selvam S, Thomas PB, Yiu SC: Tissue engineering: current and future approaches to ocular surface reconstruction. Ocul Surf 2006;4:120–136.

3 Hann LE, Tatro JB, Sullivan DA: Morphology and function of lacrimal gland acinar cells in primary culture. Invest Ophthalmol Vis Sci 1989;30:145–158.

4 Bradley ME, Lambert RW, Lambert RW, Lee LM, Mircheff AK: Isolation and subcellular fractionation analysis of acini from rabbit lacrimal glands. Invest Ophthalmol Vis Sci 1992;33:2951–2965.

5 Yoshino K, Tseng SC, Pflugfelder SC: Substrate modulation of morphology, growth, and tear protein production by cultured human lacrimal gland epithelial cells. Exp Cell Res 1995;220:138–151.
6 Selvam S, Thomas PB, Trousdale MD, Stevenson D, Schechter JE, Mircheff AK, Jacob JT, Smith RE, Yiu SC: Tissue-engineered tear secretory system: functional lacrimal gland acinar cells cultured on matrix protein-coated substrata. J Biomed Mater Res B Appl Biomater 2007;80:192–200.
7 Azuara-Blanco A, Pillai CT, Dua HS: Amniotic membrane transplantation for ocular surface reconstruction. Br J Ophthalmol 1999;83:399–402.
8 Schrader S, et al: Amniotic membrane as a carrier for lacrimal gland acinar cells. Graefes Arch Clin Exp Ophthalmol 2007;245:1699–1704.
9 Aoi T, Yae K, Nakagawa M, Ichisaka T, Okita K, Takahashi K, Chiba T, Yamanaka S: Generation of pluripotent stem cells from adult mouse liver and stomach cells. Science 2008;321:699–702.
10 Okita K, Ichisaka T, Yamanaka S: Generation of germline-competent induced pluripotent stem cells. Nature 2007;448:313–317.
11 Meller D, Tseng SC: Conjunctival epithelial cell differentiation on amniotic membrane. Invest Ophthalmol Vis Sci 1999;40:878–886.
12 Koizumi, N, Inatomi T, Quantock AJ, Fullwood NJ, Dota A, Kinoshita S: Amniotic membrane as a substrate for cultivating limbal corneal epithelial cells for autologous transplantation in rabbits. Cornea 2000;19:65–71.
13 Schwab IR: Cultured corneal epithelia for ocular surface disease. Trans Am Ophthalmol Soc 1999;97: 891–986.
14 Honavar SG, Bansal AK, Sangwan VS, Rao GN: Amniotic membrane transplantation for ocular surface reconstruction in Stevens-Johnson syndrome. Ophthalmology 2000;107:975–979.
15 Lee SH, Tseng SC: Amniotic membrane transplantation for persistent epithelial defects with ulceration. Am J Ophthalmol 1997;123:303–312.
16 Barabino S, Rolando M, Bentivoglio G, Mingari C, Zanardi S, Bellomo R, Calabria G: Role of amniotic membrane transplantation for conjunctival reconstruction in ocular-cicatrical pemphigoid. Ophthalmology 2003;110:474–480.
17 Ang LP, Tan DT, Cajucom-Uy H, Beuerman RW: Autologous cultivated conjunctival transplantation for pterygium surgery. Am J Ophthalmol 2005;139: 611–619.
18 Nakamura T, Inatomi T, Sotozono C, Amemiya T, Kanamura N, Kinoshita S: Transplantation of cultivated autologous oral mucosal epithelial cells in patients with severe ocular surface disorders. Br J Ophthalmol 2004;88:1280–1284.
19 Lewis ML, Moriarity DM, Campbell PS: Use of microgravity bioreactors for development of an in vitro rat salivary gland cell culture model. J Cell Biochem 1993;51:265–273.
20 Becker JL, Prewett TL, Spaulding GF, Goodwin TJ: Three-dimensional growth and differentiation of ovarian tumor cell line in high aspect rotating-wall vessel: morphologic and embryologic considerations. J Cell Biochem 1993;51:283–289.
21 Goodwin, TJ, Jessup JM, Wolf DA: Morphologic differentiation of colon carcinoma cell lines HT-29 and HT-29KM in rotating-wall vessels. In Vitro Cell Dev Biol 1992;28A:47–60.
22 Hatfill, SJ, Margolis LB, Duray PH: In vitro maintenance of normal and pathological human salivary gland tissue in a NASA-designed rotating wall vessel bioreactor. Cell Vision 1996;3:5.
23 Schrader S, Kremling C, Klinger M, Laqua H, Geerling G: Cultivation of lacrimal gland acinar cells in a microgravity environment. Br J Ophthalmol 2009; 93:1121–1125.
24 Pellegrini G, Traverso CE, Franzi AT, Zingirian M, Cancedda R, De Luca M: Long-term restoration of damaged corneal surfaces with autologous cultivated corneal epithelium. Lancet 1997;349:990–993.
25 Schrader S, Notara M, Beaconsfield M, Tuft S, Geerling G, Daniels JT: Conjunctival epithelial cells maintain stem cell properties after long-term culture and cryopreservation. Regen Med 2009;4:677–687.
26 Kishi T, Takao T, Fujita K, Taniguchi H: Clonal proliferation of multipotent stem/progenitor cells in the neonatal and adult salivary glands. Biochem Biophys Res Commun 2006;340:544–552.
27 Holland AM, Gonez LJ, Harrison LC: Progenitor cells in the adult pancreas. Diabetes Metab Res Rev 2004;20:13–27.
28 Zhang YQ, Kritzik M, Sarvetnick N: Identification and expansion of pancreatic stem/progenitor cells. J Cell Mol Med 2005;9:331–344.
29 Zoukhri D, Fix A, Alroy J, Kublin CL: Mechanisms of murine lacrimal gland repair after experimentally induced inflammation. Invest Ophthalmol Vis Sci 2008;49:4399–4406.
30 Geerling G, Sieg P, Bastian GO, Laqua H: Transplantation of the autologous submandibular gland for most severe cases of keratoconjunctivitis sicca. Ophthalmology 1998;105:327–335.
31 Revoltella RP, Papini S, Rosellini A, Michelini M: Epithelial stem cells of the eye surface. Cell Prolif 2007;40:445–461.

32 Meller, D, Dabul V, Tseng SC: Expansion of conjunctival epithelial progenitor cells on amniotic membrane. Exp Eye Res 2002;74:537–545.

33 Meller, D, Pires RT, Tseng SC: Ex vivo preservation and expansion of human limbal epithelial stem cells on amniotic membrane cultures. Br J Ophthalmol 2002;86:463–471.

34 Tsai, RJ, Li LM, Chen JK: Reconstruction of damaged corneas by transplantation of autologous limbal epithelial cells. N Engl J Med 2000;343:86–93.

35 Matsumoto T, Mooney DJ: Cell instructive polymers. Adv Biochem Eng Biotechnol 2006;102:113–137.

Stefan Schrader, MD
Cells for Sight Transplantation and Research Programme
Department of Ocular Biology and Therapeutics, UCL Institute of Ophthalmology
11–43 Bath Street, EC1V 9EL London (UK)
Tel. +44 207 608 6996, Fax +44 207 608 6887, E-Mail mail@stefanschrader.de

Brewitt H (ed): Research Projects in Dry Eye Syndrome.
Dev Ophthalmol. Basel, Karger, 2010, vol 45, pp 57–70

Midterm Results of Cultivated Autologous and Allogeneic Limbal Epithelial Transplantation in Limbal Stem Cell Deficiency

Mikk Pauklin · Thomas A. Fuchsluger · Henrike Westekemper · Klaus-P. Steuhl · Daniel Meller

Department of Ophthalmology, University of Duisburg-Essen, Essen, Germany

Abstract

Background: Limbal stem cell deficiency (LSCD) leads to growth of abnormal fibro-vascular pannus tissue onto the corneal surface as well as chronic inflammation and impaired vision. Our aim was to investigate the clinical outcome of ocular surface reconstruction in LSCD using limbal epithelial cells expanded on amniotic membrane (AM). **Methods:** Forty-four eyes of 38 patients (27 male, 11 female) with total (n = 32) or partial (n = 12) LSCD were treated by transplantation of autologous (n = 30) or allogeneic (n = 14) limbal epithelial cells expanded on intact AM. LSCD was caused by chemical and thermal burns (n = 22), pterygium (n = 9), congenital aniridia (n = 6), tumor excision (n = 2), perforating eye injury, mitomycin C, epidermolysis bullosa, bilateral graft-versus-host disease and chlamydial conjunctivitis (each n = 1). **Results:** Mean follow-up time was 28.5 ± 14.9 months. The corneal surface could be reconstructed to full stability in 30 (68%), and clear central cornea was achieved in 37 (84%) eyes. Grafting was significantly more successful in eyes treated by autologous than by allogeneic transplantation (76.7 vs. 50%, $p < 0.05$). The corneal surface could be successfully restored in 10 (83.3%) eyes with partial LSCD and in 20 (63.3%) eyes with total LSCD. Visual acuity (VA) increased significantly in 32 (73%) eyes, was stable in 10 (23%) eyes and decreased in 2 (4%) eyes. Mean VA increased significantly ($p < 0.0001$), from preoperative 1.7 ± 0.9 logMAR (20/1,000) to 0.9 ± 0.7 logMAR (20/160). VA increased significantly after both autologous ($p < 0.0001$) and allogeneic transplantation ($p < 0.005$). **Conclusions:** In most patients with LSCD, transplantation of limbal epithelium cultivated on intact AM restores the corneal surface and results in significantly increased VA.

M.P. and T.A.F. should be considered first authors.

Several studies have pointed to the limbus as a location of corneal epithelial stem cells, and have characterized its role in corneal epithelial homeostasis [1, 2]. These cells may be destroyed by local and systemic conditions [3], and the resulting limbal stem cell deficiency (LSCD) is characterized by the growth of abnormal fibrovascular pannus tissue onto the corneal surface as well as chronic inflammation and impaired vision [4, 5].

In patients with LSCD, perforating keratoplasty has a limited success rate because no stem cells are transferred and the underlying cause of corneal vascularization and epithelial instability remains untreated [6, 7]. In partial LSCD, the transplantation of amniotic membrane (AM) alone may be effective, probably because it supports proliferation of the patients' own remaining stem cells [8]. Sequential sector conjunctival epitheliectomy – wherein pannus covering a sector of the cornea and limbus is removed and prevented from crossing the limbus until the denuded surface is covered by corneal epithelium derived cells – may be used in cases of partial LSCD with a thin pannus [9]. In severe cases, replenishment of the stem cell pool by transplantation of limbal stem cells is necessary [10]. Since the first transplantation of a limbal rim in 1989 [11], various treatment modalities of LSCD have been developed. The clinical outcomes of more than 600 eyes with LSCD treated by transplantation of autologous or allogeneic limbus have recently been summarized in a literature review [12]. Initially, relatively large pieces of autologous [11] or allogeneic [13–15] limbal tissue were transplanted, often simultaneously with perforating [16] or lamellar [17] keratoplasty. Although short-term results were promising, graft rejection occurred rather frequently [18–20]. Graft survival rates declined from 40–54% after 1 year, to 33% after 2 years, and 27% after 3 years [19, 21]. The transplanted limbal tissue was vascularized, highly antigenic, contained Langerhans cells and was thus often rejected [22, 23]. Even under topical and systemic immunosuppression, a 36% endothelial rejection rate has been reported for simultaneous allogeneic limbal and perforating corneal transplantations [16]. Human leukocyte antigen matching seemed to be beneficial [18, 20], but the outcome remained poor [21]. Patients with Stevens-Johnson syndrome, dry eye, corneal keratinization, eyelid abnormalities or allogeneic limbal transplantation had especially poor surgical outcomes [21].

To overcome these shortcomings, tissue engineering by means of ex vivo expansion of undifferentiated limbal epithelium was developed [24]. Its main advantages are minimal iatrogenic damage to the donor site due to a small biopsy and the possibility of avoiding immunosuppression by using autologous tissue [25–27]. Since the first report [24], different cultivation methods have been developed and the clinical results of about 200 eyes with LSCD have been reported [for reviews, see 4, 12]. Although the method has recently gained popularity, strong evidence of its effectiveness is lacking due to a relatively small number of reported patients [4, 12].

In the present study, we report the clinical outcome of 44 eyes with total or partial LSCD that were treated by transplantation of ex vivo on intact AM-expanded autologous as well as allogeneic limbal epithelium.

Materials and Methods

This study was approved by the Ethics Committee of the University Duisburg-Essen. All research was conducted in accordance with the tenets of the Declaration of Helsinki (1989 version).

Patients

Forty-four eyes of 38 patients (27 male and 11 female) with total (n = 32) or partial (n = 12) LSCD were treated during the chronic phase of the disease or at least 12 months after the initial trauma. Transplantation of cultivated limbal epithelium (TCLE) on intact AM was performed between 2003 and 2008 at the University Eye Clinic in Essen. Consecutive cases with a follow-up time of at least 9 months were included in the study. LSCD was diagnosed by clinical examination using recognized diagnostic criteria: epithelial fragility, hyperpermeability of the corneal epithelium, superficial corneal neovascularization, and growth of pannus tissue onto the corneal surface [28]. Conjunctivalization and the presence of goblet cells on the corneal surface was confirmed in all cases through impression cytology [29]. Age at surgery was 45.4 ± 17.4 years (mean ± SD, range 6–80 years). We were able to transplant autologous tissue from the less- or unaffected fellow eye in 30 eyes. The mean age at surgery in this group was 47.4 ± 20.1 (range 8–79) years. Allogeneic tissue from either living relatives (n = 4) or deceased donors (n = 10) was used in the remaining 14 eyes, mostly in patients with bilateral LSCD. The mean age at surgery was 41.1 ± 8 (range 28–56) years. The etiology of LSCD comprised chemical and thermal burns (n = 22), extensive recurrent pterygium (n = 9), congenital aniridia (n = 6), tumor excision (n = 2), perforating injury, mitomycin-C-induced LSCD, epidermolysis bullosa, bilateral graft-versus-host disease and chlamydial conjunctivitis (each n = 1).

Ex vivo Expansion of Limbal Epithelial Cells on AM

All donors underwent serological testing to detect the human immunodeficiency virus, human hepatitis virus types B and C, and syphilis prior to tissue donation. Written informed consent was obtained from all donors and recipients. AM was obtained as described elsewhere [30]. At least 2 biopsy pieces measuring 1 × 2 mm were harvested from the corneal limbus in topical anesthesia. Eyes from deceased multiorgan donors were obtained within 24 h of brain death. The cultivation method of limbal epithelial cells has been reported elsewhere [31, 32]. Briefly, the limbal pieces were treated for 7 min with 1.2 U/ml Dispase II in Hank's balanced salt solution at 37°C. After a rinse with PBS, the limbal pieces were placed on the epithelial side of intact AM fastened onto a culture insert, as reported earlier [33], and cultured in the previously described supplemental hormonal epithelial medium [25]. The medium contained equal volumes of HEPES-buffered Dulbecco's modified Eagle's medium containing bicarbonate and Ham's F12 (all from Invitrogen, N.Y., USA), and was supplemented with 10% autologous serum, 0.5% dimethyl sulfoxide, 2 ng/ml mouse epidermal growth factor, 5 mg/ml insulin, 5 mg/ml transferrin, 5 ng/ml selenium, 0.5 mg/ml hydrocortisone, 30 ng/ml cholera toxin A subunit, 50 mg/ml gentamicin and 1.25 mg/ml amphotericin B (all from Sigma-Aldrich, St. Louis, Mo., USA). Cultures were submerged in growth medium and cultured at 37°C under 5% carbon dioxide and 95% air. The medium was changed every 2–3 days. Air-lifting described by several groups [33, 34] was not used to avoid cell differentiation. No feeder cells were used. Outgrowth was monitored and documented using phase contrast microscopy (Eclipse TE2000-S, Nikon Corporation, Tokyo, Japan). Transplantation was performed after approximately 14 days.

Surgical Procedures

All procedures were performed under general anesthesia by 2 experienced surgeons (D.M./K.-P.S). After 360-degree conjunctival peritomy and recession of the bulbar conjunctiva, the fibrovascular pannus was carefully dissected from the corneal surface. The cultivated limbal epithelial cell layer on AM was transferred onto the bare sclera and corneal stroma, and secured to the underlying episclera and limbus with interrupted and to the adjacent conjunctiva with mattress-like 10–0 nylon sutures. A second preserved AM that served as a patch was secured with interrupted 8–0 vicryl (Ethicon, Norderstedt, Germany) sutures to the surrounding bulbar conjunctiva.

Postoperative Treatment

Ptosis was induced in all patients within the first week after surgery by injecting 30 units Dysport® (Ipsen Pharma GmbH, Ettlingen, Germany) into the musculus levator palpebrae to reduce friction of the upper eyelid upon the graft [35]. Postoperative medications included preservative-free 3% ofloxacine (Floxal EDO®, Mann Pharma, Berlin, Germany), preservative-free sodium hyaluronate eye drops (Hylocommod, Ursapharm, Saarbrücken, Germany) and 20% autologous serum eye drops (5 times per day for at least 12 months). Additionally, 1% preservative-free dexamethasone eye drops (Dexasine SE, Alcon Pharma, Freiburg, Germany) were applied and tapered off after 3 months. All patients that received allografts, except 2, were treated with cyclosporin A (Sandimmun, Novartis Deutschland, Nürnberg, Germany) as systemic immunosuppression (cyclosporin A 100 mg twice per day for 12–15 months according to cyclosporin blood level). One patient received 360–720 mg mycophenolate mofetil (Myfortic®, Novartis Deutschland) twice per day for 18 months because cyclosporin A was not tolerated, and the remaining patient was not treated by any immunosuppressive regime.

Outcome Evaluation

Pre- and postoperative examinations involved determination of visual acuity (VA), slit-lamp examination, photo documentation and fluorescein staining to assess ocular surface integrity. Restoration of ocular surface integrity was considered the major outcome measure, as it is directly affected by transplantation of cultivated limbal epithelium. Improvement in VA was regarded as the minor outcome measure.

A scoring system and numeric coding enabled statistical analysis of the outcome [36]. Successful grafting (1) was defined as a procedure that resulted in an entirely clear, smooth and stable corneal surface, with persistent epithelial closure and without invasion of pannus tissue or recurrence of superficial corneal vascularization during the follow-up period. Grafting was considered partially successful (2) in cases of recurrent defects of the corneal epithelium detected by fluorescein staining or peripheral superficial neovascularization in no more than 1 quadrant, but with remaining central corneal transparency. Failed grafting (3) was defined as the presence of therapy-resistant persistent epithelial defects, extensive superficial neovascularization in more than 1 quadrant and/or loss of central corneal transparency caused by recurrent growth of pannus tissue or a pterygium onto the corneal surface [37]. A change of ≥2 lines in final VA (0.1 logMAR steps) compared to preoperative VA was considered significant. VA 'hand motion at 1-ft distance' was calculated as 2.3 logMAR (20/4,000), 'counting fingers at 1-ft distance' as 2.0 LogMAR (20/2,000) [38].

Statistical Analysis

Statistical analysis was performed using SPSS for Windows 16.0 (SPSS, Chicago, Ill., USA). Values of $p < 0.05$ were considered to be statistically significant. Independent-samples t tests were used to compare the demographic data, preoperative VA, final VA, follow-up times and VA outcome with ocular surface restoration rates in different treatment groups. Paired-sample t tests were used to compare preoperative and final VA in different treatment groups. Kaplan-Meier survival analysis and Cox regression analysis were used to analyze survival and failure risk of cultivated limbal grafts.

Results

Outcome of Corneal Surface Reconstruction

Mean ± SD follow-up was 28.5 ± 14.9 (9–73) months, and did not differ significantly between treatment groups. Patients with total LSCD were significantly ($p < 0.0001$) younger (39.4 ± 12.4 years) than patients with partial LSCD (61.3 ± 19.0 years). Corneal surface reconstruction was completely successful in 30 (68.2%), partially successful in 7 (15.9%) and failed in 7 (15.9%) eyes (fig. 1, 2a; table 1). A stable central corneal epithelium and a clear visual axis could be restored in 37 (84.1%) eyes. Almost all patients reported improved subjective symptoms, like pain and sensation of irritation, in conjunction with ocular surface regeneration.

Grafting was significantly more successful in eyes treated by autologous than by allogeneic transplantation (76.7 vs. 50%, $p < 0.05$; fig. 2b). A stable central corneal surface could be restored in 27 (90%) eyes treated by autologous and in 10 (71.4%) eyes treated by allogeneic transplantation of intact-AM-cultivated limbal epithelium (TCLE). Allogeneic grafting had a 1.95-fold higher risk of partial or complete graft failure ($p < 0.05$). Corneal surface could be successfully restored in 10 (83.3%) eyes with partial LSCD and in 20 (63.3%) eyes with total LSCD (fig. 2c).

The etiology of LSCD had an impact on the efficacy of the procedure (fig. 2d). LSCD after a chemical or thermal burn could successfully be treated in 14 (63.6%) eyes. Again, autologous transplantation was significantly more successful than allogeneic grafting (75 vs. 33.3%, $p < 0.05$). A stable corneal surface was restored in 10 (90%) eyes treated by autologous TCLE for treatment of partial LSCD caused by excision of pterygium or a conjunctival tumor. LSCD caused by congenital aniridia was in all cases treated by allogeneic TCLE and showed a successful outcome in 3 (50%) eyes. One patient died from lung cancer 28 months after limbal stem cell transplantation.

VA Outcome

VA increased significantly in 32 (72.7%), was stable in 10 (22.7%) and decreased in 2 (4.5%) eyes. Mean VA increased significantly ($p < 0.0001$) from preoperative 1.7 ± 0.9 logMAR (20/1,000) to 0.9 ± 0.7 logMAR (20/160). On average, 8.7 lines (0.1 logMAR steps) were gained after therapy (table 2). As expected, significantly more eyes with successful or partially successful TCLE ($p < 0.05$; $p < 0.01$ respectively) improved in VA than eyes with failed TCLE. Eyes with preoperative VA of hand motion or counting fingers had the most significant benefit from therapy (fig. 3a). Nine (20.5%) eyes showed a 2- to 9-line, 6 (13.6%) eyes a 10- to 14-line, and 17 (38.6%) eyes a 15- to 20-line improvement in VA (fig. 3b).

Both the mean preoperative and final VA were significantly better in the autologous transplantation group than in the allogeneic group ($p < 0.05$ and < 0.0001, respectively). After autologous transplantation, VA increased in 21 (70%) eyes. Mean VA increased significantly from 1.6 ± 1 (20/800) to 0.6 ± 0.5 (20/80) logMAR

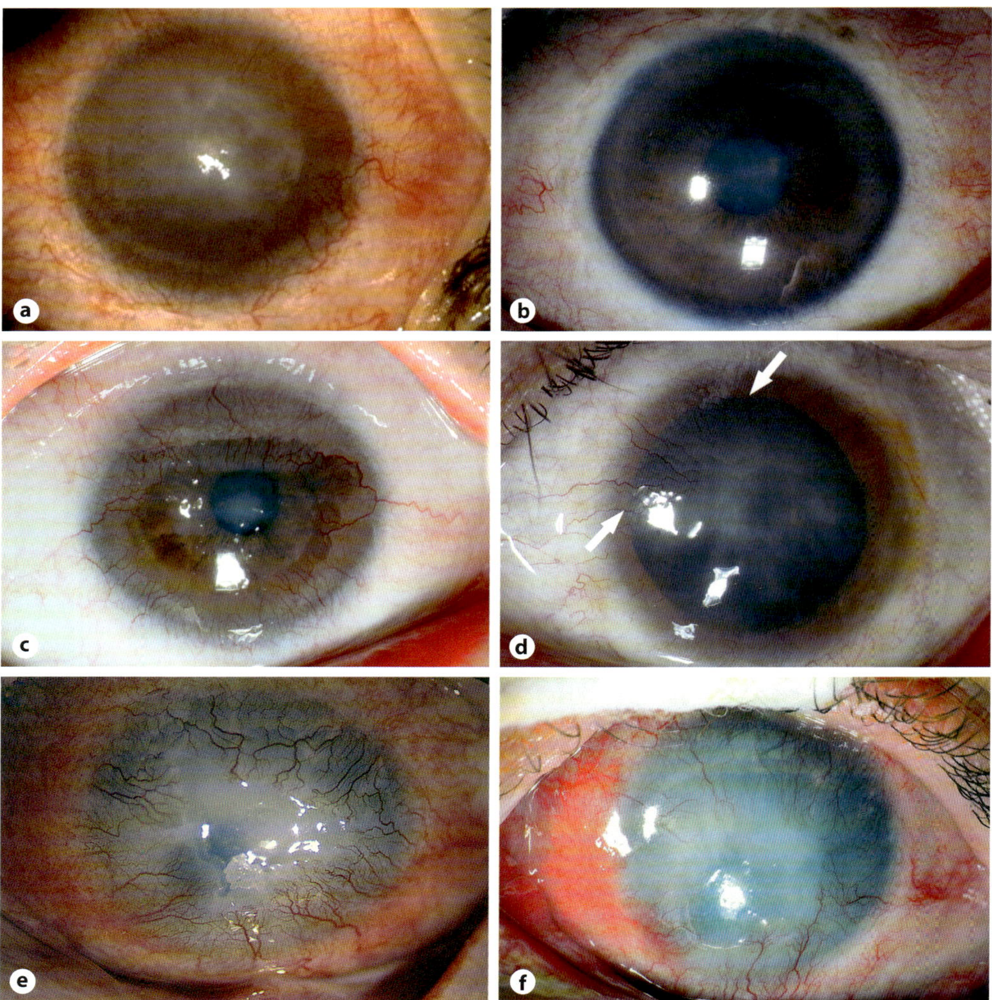

Fig. 1. Outcome of corneal surface reconstruction. **a**, **b** Successful transplantation of cultivated autologous limbal epithelium for the treatment of total LSCD caused by a chemical burn. Preoperatively, the complete corneal surface was covered by fibrovascular pannus tissue and VA was reduced to hand motion (2.3 LogMAR) (**a**). The ocular surface is stable, the cornea clear and VA increased to 0.4 logMAR 73 months after transplantation of cultivated limbal epithelium (**b**). **c**, **d** Sample of a partially successful transplantation of allogeneic cultivated limbal epithelium for the treatment of total bilateral LSCD after a chemical burn. Preoperatively, a 360-degree vascularization of the cornea and VA was reduced to counting fingers (2.0 logMAR) (**c**). Recurrence of superficial vascularization (arrows) was noted in the upper-left quadrant 1 month after surgery, but had not progressed to the visual axis 12 months after surgery and VA increased to 0.1 logMAR (**d**). **e**, **f** Sample of a failed allogeneic transplantation for the treatment of total bilateral LSCD after a severe chemical burn. **e** Preoperatively, the cornea was vascularized and scarred, VA hand motion (2.3 logMAR). **f** LSCD reappeared 1 month after surgery and led to revascularization of the cornea 18 months after surgery.

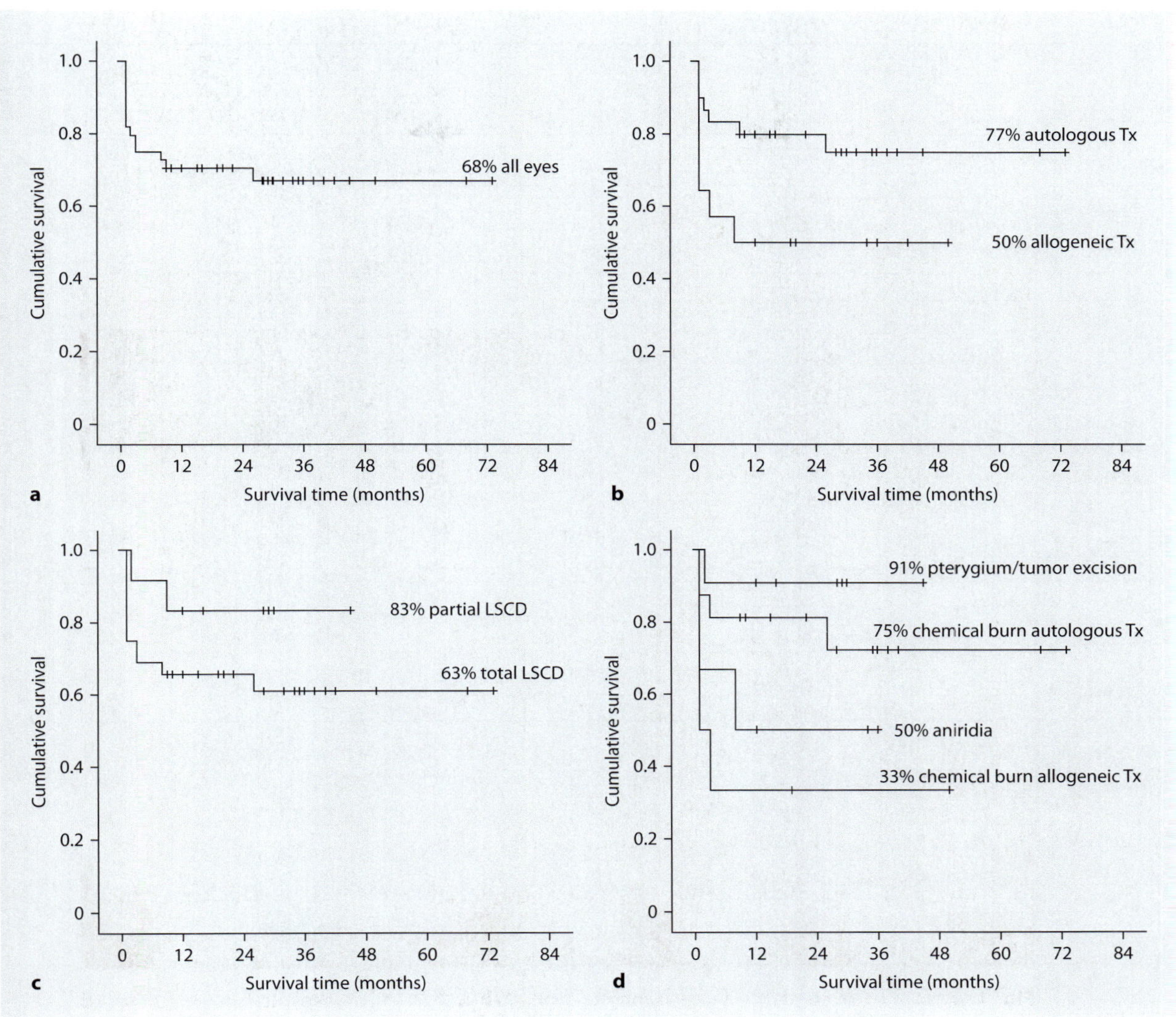

Fig. 2. Kaplan-Meier analysis of stable corneal surface survival. First appearance of corneal surface instability, corneal neovascularization or pannus invasion that finally led to a partial or complete failure of the procedure was defined as event. **a** Survival analysis of all treated eyes (n = 44). **b** Eyes treated by autologous (n = 30) transplantation (Tx) showed a significantly higher ($p < 0.05$) survival rate than eyes treated by allogeneic transplantation (n = 14). **c** Partial LSCD (n = 12) had a better outcome rate than total LSCD (n = 32). **d** Graft survival differed according to the etiology of LSCD.

($p < 0.0001$). VA increased in 9 (64.3%) eyes treated with allogeneic TCLE. Mean VA increased significantly from 2.3 ± 0.3 to 1.4 ± 0.7 logMAR ($p < 0.005$). VA increased in significantly more eyes with total LSCD (87.5%) than in eyes with partial LSCD (33.3%, $p < 0.005$). Eyes with total LSCD also gained significantly more (12 lines) lines on average than eyes with partial LSCD (2 lines; $p < 0.0001$).

Table 1. Outcome of corneal surface restoration in different groups,

	Eyes, n	Successful		Partially successful		Failed	
		eyes, n	%	eyes, n	%	eyes, n	%
All treated eyes	44	30	68.2	7	15.9	7	15.9
Type of donor tissue							
Autologous transplantations	30	23	76.7	4	13.3	3	10.0
Allogeneic transplantations	14	7	50.0	3	21.4	4	28.6
Extent of LSCD							
Total LSCD	32	20	62.5	6	18.8	6	18.8
Partial LSCD	12	10	83.3	1	8.3	1	8.3
Etiology of LSCD							
CMB (all)	22	14	63.6	5	22.7	3	13.6
CMB (autologous)	16	12	75.0	3	18.8	1	6.3
CMB (allogeneic)	6	2	33.3	2	33.3	2	33.3
Pterygium/tumor excision	11	10	90.9	0	0.0	1	9.1
Aniridia	6	3	50.0	1	16.7	2	33.3

CMB = Chemical/thermal burn.

Etiology of LSCD had a significant impact on VA outcome ($p = 0.001$). Eyes treated after a chemical or thermal burn had the best VA outcome. VA increased in 18 (81.8%) of these eyes and mean VA increased by 13 lines ($p < 0.0001$). Autologous transplantation for chemical or thermal burns resulted in a significantly higher number of eyes with improved VA ($p < 0.05$). Additionally, the improvement in VA of this group was significantly higher in comparison to allogeneic transplantation ($p < 0.005$). After autologous transplantation for chemical/thermal burns, VA increased in 15 (93.8%) eyes, the mean increase was highly significant ($p < 0.0001$) and the average eye gained 16 lines. In contrast, after allogeneic transplantation, VA increased in 3 (50%) eyes by an average of 6 lines. VA increased in 2 (22.2%) eyes with pterygium, although mean VA did not change significantly due to comparatively good preoperative VA. VA increased in 4 (66.7%) eyes with congenital aniridia and by an average of 6 lines.

Additional Procedures

During the follow-up period, 11 eyes received perforating keratoplasty (concomitant, n = 3; subsequent, n = 8), and 5 had intraocular lenses implanted. Eleven eyes with a partially successful outcome received subconjunctival bevacizumab (Avastin, Roche,

Table 2. VA outcome in different treatment groups

	Preoperative VA (logMAR)		Final VA (logMAR)		Mean improved 0.1 logMAR	Paired-samples t test	
	mean ± SD	median	mean ± SD	median		p value	95% CI
All treated eyes	1.7±0.9	2.3	0.9±0.7	0.7	9	<0.0001	0.6–1.1
Type of donor tissue							
Autologous transplantations	1.6±1	2.3	0.6±0.5	0.5	10	<0.0001	0.6–1.3
Allogeneic transplantations	2.3±0.3	2.3	1.4±0.7	1.3	7	<0.005	0.3–1.2
Extent of LSCD							
Total LSCD	2.2±0.2	2.3	1.0±0.6	0.8	12	<0.0001	0.7 to 1.1
Partial LSCD	0.5±0.6	0.3	0.3±0.3	0.2	2	>0.05	−0.1 to 0.[illegible]
Etiology of LSCD							
CMB (all)	2.2±0.3	2.3	0.9±0.6	0.7	13	<0.0001	1.0 to 1.6
CMB (autologous)	2.3±0	2.3	0.7±0.5	0.6	16	<0.0001	1.3 to 1.8
CMB (allogeneic)	2±0.5	2.2	1.2±0.9	1	6	0.07	−0.1 to 1.[illegible]
Pterygium/ tumor excision	0.3±0.2	0.2	0.3±0.3	0.3	0	>0.05	− 0.1 to 0.[illegible]
Aniridia	2.3±0.1	2.3	1.7±0.5	1.5	6	0.06	−0.1 to 1.1

CMB = Chemical/thermal burn.

Mannheim, Germany) injections to inhibit further progression of corneal neovascularization. All patients who received subconjunctival bevacizumab injections during the follow-up period were classified as partially successful or failed procedures, despite the fact that some of these patients had an intact corneal surface without any superficial vascularization on the last examination. Therefore, bevacizumab injections did not distort the success rate of limbal epithelial transplantation.

Complications

Postoperative complications included 1 case of large but self-resolving bleeding beneath the AM sheet. In 2 cases, corneal perforation developed. One case was caused by preoperative corneal thinning with formation of a descemetocele and the other by preoperative corneal thinning combined with trichiasis. Both were treated with a tectonic or optical perforating keratoplasty.

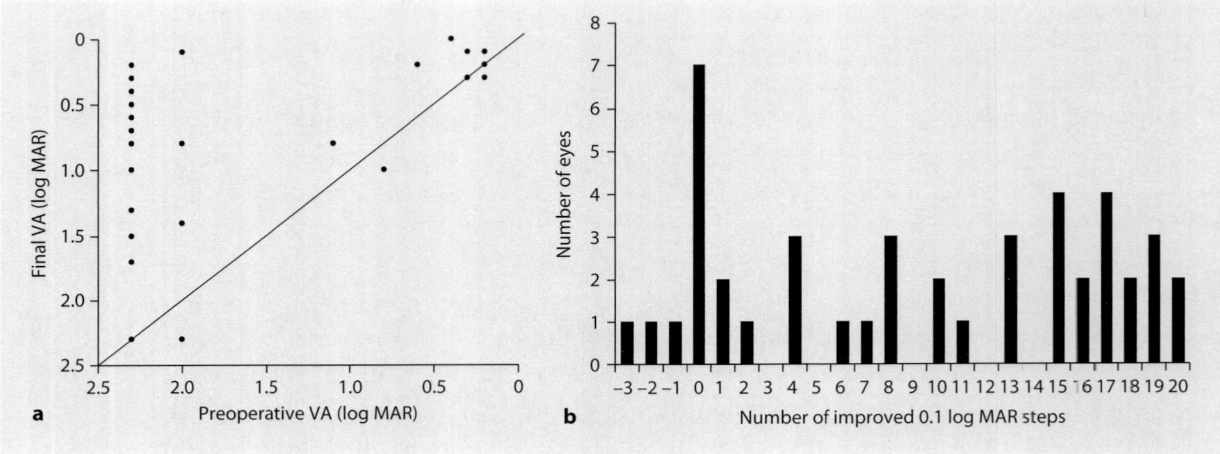

Fig. 3. VA outcome of all treated patients. **a** Scatter plot presenting preoperative and final VA in logMAR of all patients. Dots above the line represent improved VA, dots on the line represent eyes with stable VA, and below the line decreased VA. The greater the distance from the line, the more substantial the change in VA. Eyes with identical preoperative and final VA are presented as single dots. Note the inverted orientation of scales due to LogMAR presentation. **b** Number of patients that gained or lost a certain number of lines (0.1 logMAR steps) in VA after therapy.

Acute limbal graft rejection with engorged limbal vessels, impairment of ocular surface integrity and an acute advancement of conjunctival tissue onto the reconstructed corneal surface [13] was noted 27 months after a partially successful allogeneic transplantation in 1 eye, but stabilized after local and systemic administration of steroids. Chronic corneal and limbal graft failure/rejection represent the cases of unfavorable outcome, as described above. Eleven (78.6%) of 14 eyes that were finally graded as partially successful procedure or failure showed signs of corneal surface instability within the first 3 months after surgery, 8 eyes (57.1%) within the first month, 1 (7.1%) within the second month, and 2 (14.3%) within the third month. This indicates that the ocular surface remained stable in most eyes where the limbal stem cell population was initially successfully restored (fig. 2).

Discussion

Our study presents the clinical outcome of 44 eyes with LSCD treated by autologous or allogeneic TCLE. The patents described here form one of the largest groups of LSCD patients, to date, treated by transplantation of cultivated limbal epithelium. Stable corneal surface was restored in 68%, a stable central corneal surface in 84%, and VA increased in 73% of all treated eyes. Since the population was rather heterogeneous and the outcome varied between patients, the mean success rate does not have a high predictive power. The formation of subgroups according to the source of donor tissue, and the extent and etiology of LSCD, allowed us to evaluate the impact of different factors on the outcome. Analysis of these homogenous subgroups yielded, despite the relatively small number of patients in each group, solid statistical evidence for the effectiveness of the used treatment method and the impact of different factors on the outcome. These data should have a higher value for the clinician and should help by the selection of appropriate therapeutics and the prediction of the outcome.

As in previous reports [21, 39], but contrary to one recent report [40], autologous transplantation had a significantly better visual outcome, a higher corneal surface restoration rate and a 2-fold lower risk for a partial or total graft failure. We therefore suggest that autologous tissue should be preferred to allogeneic limbal tissue whenever possible. The reason for failure in the unsuccessful cases may have been too few transferred stem cells or their destruction after transplantation. Chronic rejection might also have been a reason for the poorer outcome of eyes treated by allogeneic transplantation [21]. The etiology and extent of LSCD had a significant impact on the outcome. As expected, partial LSCD had a better ocular surface restoration rate than total LSCD. Due to the complexity of the method, transplantation of cultivated limbal epithelium should be used for treatment of partial LSCD only in the most severe cases, when all other conventional therapy methods have failed. Our results suggest that in these selected cases, transplantation of cultivated limbal epithelium has an excellent outcome. The etiology of LSCD also had a significant impact on the outcome. The highest improvement in VA was achieved in patients with LSCD after a chemical or thermal burn, especially if treated by autologous transplantation. Almost all of these patients had a preoperative VA that could be described as hand motion, but which improved in almost all cases above 20/200. The reason for the favorable outcome in eyes with a chemical burn may be the one-time trauma that caused LSCD. Eyes affected by continuous processes like cicatrical pemphigoid or Stevens-Johnson syndrome have a significantly worse outcome [41]. The management of aniridic keratopathy was in most cases successful, but the visual improvement was limited because of the other ocular anomalies caused by the *Pax6* gene mutation [42]. The herein reported data may help the clinicians to assess the prognosis of a particular patient and to decide between different treatments.

As reported earlier [25, 32, 33, 43, 44], we used a completely xenobiotic-free culture system. The system is based on autologous serum as supplement to the growth medium avoiding fetal bovine serum – an important aspect in the current safety-related discussion regarding eventual transmission of Creutzfeldt-Jakob disease and shows a similar efficacy to fetal bovine serum [45]. The avoidance of airlifting and the use of intact AM as culture substrate, allowed us to transplant relatively undifferentiated limbal cells without the use of mouse 3T3 fibroblast feeder layers [46]. In addition, the transplanted basement membrane of AM served as basement membrane replacement. Postoperative treatment was directed to protect and support the healing ocular surface. It involved an AM patch and application of autologous serum eye drops to enhance reepithelization as well as the induction of ptosis to protect the transplanted cells [35].

In this report, diagnosis of LSCD was established based on well-recognized clinical symptoms in combination with fluorescein staining and impression cytology. In the excised pannus, we have previously found a conjunctival expression pattern of tissue-specific keratins as well as membrane-associated mucins and an increased expression of inflammatory markers confirming the LSCD diagnosis. We have also previously shown that the regenerated and stable corneal surfaces of patients treated by this procedure have indeed regained a corneal phenotype [31, 32]. In contrast to previous reports [20], we distinguished between successful and partially successful procedures. Eyes with focal peripheral ingrowth of pannus and peripheral superficial vascularization should be considered only partially successful, as the limbal barrier was not completely restored, although the procedure was in most cases accompanied by improvements in VA and subjective symptoms.

We considered restoration of an intact corneal surface a major outcome measure as it depends directly on the restoration of the limbal stem cell population. In our opinion, additional procedures that were performed during the follow-up period did not distort the corneal surface restoration rate. Previous reports have shown that keratoplasty succeeds only in eyes with a restored stem cell population [6, 7]. Improvement in VA was considered a minor outcome measure as it did not depend solely on the restoration of a stable corneal surface, but also on the clarity of other optical media, like the corneal stroma, the lens, and vitreous and retinal and optic nerve function. Therefore, additional procedures like keratoplasty and intraocular lens implantations that were performed in some of the patients had an impact of the final visual outcome.

In conclusion, our results show that transplantation of intact-AM-cultivated limbal epithelium is safe, restores a stable corneal surface in most patients with LSCD, and is often accompanied by significant visual improvement. Further studies should address whether our results can be confirmed in a larger population.

Acknowledgments

Partially supported by the Estonian Scientific Foundation (grant No. 5832), Deutsche Ophthalmologische Gesellschaft (German Society of Ophthalmology), Deutsche Forschungsgemeinschaft (German Research Foundation, Bonn, ME 1623/3-1), and Forschungsförderung AG Trockenes Auge, Berlin, Germany.

References

1 Cotsarelis G, Cheng SZ, Dong G, Sun TT, Lavker RM: Existence of slow-cycling limbal epithelial basal cells that can be preferentially stimulated to proliferate: implications on epithelial stem cells. Cell 1989;57:201.

2 Schermer A, Galvin S, Sun TT: Differentiation-related expression of a major 64K corneal keratin in vivo and in culture suggests limbal location of corneal epithelial stem cells. J Cell Biol 1986;103:49.

3 Holland EJ, Schwartz GS: The evolution of epithelial transplantation for severe ocular surface disease and a proposed classification system. Cornea 1996;15:549.

4 Shortt AJ, Secker GA, Notara MD, et al: Transplantation of ex vivo cultured limbal epithelial stem cells: a review of techniques and clinical results. Surv Ophthalmol 2007;52:483.

5 Dua HS, Forrester JV: The corneoscleral limbus in human corneal epithelial wound healing. Am J Ophthalmol 1990;110:646.

6 Sangwan VS, Fernandes M, Bansal AK, Vemuganti GK, Rao GN: Early results of penetrating keratoplasty following limbal stem cell transplantation. Indian J Ophthalmol 2005;53:31.

7 Dua HS, Rahman I, Jayaswal R, Said DG: Combined limbal and corneal grafts: should we or should we not? Clin Experiment Ophthalmol 2008;36:497.

8 Anderson DF, Ellies P, Pires RT, Tseng SC: Amniotic membrane transplantation for partial limbal stem cell deficiency. Br J Ophthalmol 2001;85:567.

9 Dua HS, Gomes JA, Singh A: Corneal epithelial wound healing. Br J Ophthalmol 1994;78:401.

10 Tseng SC, Prabhasawat P, Barton K, Gray T, Meller D: Amniotic membrane transplantation with or without limbal allografts for corneal surface reconstruction in patients with limbal stem cell deficiency. Arch Ophthalmol 1998;116:431.

11 Kenyon KR, Tseng SC: Limbal autograft transplantation for ocular surface disorders. Ophthalmology 1989;96:709.

12 Cauchi PA, Ang GS, Azuara-Blanco A, Burr JM: A systematic literature review of surgical interventions for limbal stem cell deficiency in humans. Am J Ophthalmol 2008;146:251.

13 Tsai RJ, Tseng SC: Human allograft limbal transplantation for corneal surface reconstruction. Cornea 1994;13:389.

14 Holland EJ: Epithelial transplantation for the management of severe ocular surface disease. Trans Am Ophthalmol Soc 1996;94:677.

15 Tsubota K, Satake Y, Kaido M, et al: Treatment of severe ocular-surface disorders with corneal epithelial stem-cell transplantation. N Engl J Med 1999;340:1697.

16 Shimazaki J, Maruyama F, Shimmura S, Fujishima H, Tsubota K: Immunologic rejection of the central graft after limbal allograft transplantation combined with penetrating keratoplasty. Cornea 2001;20:149.

17 Yao YF, Zhang B, Zhou P, Jiang JK: Autologous limbal grafting combined with deep lamellar keratoplasty in unilateral eye with severe chemical or thermal burn at late stage. Ophthalmology 2002;109:2011.

18 Rao SK, Rajagopal R, Sitalakshmi G, Padmanabhan P: Limbal allografting from related live donors for corneal surface reconstruction. Ophthalmology 1999;106:822.

19 Ilari L, Daya SM: Long-term outcomes of keratolimbal allograft for the treatment of severe ocular surface disorders. Ophthalmology 2002;109:1278.

20 Reinhard T, Spelsberg H, Henke L, et al: Long-term results of allogeneic penetrating limbo-keratoplasty in total limbal stem cell deficiency. Ophthalmology 2004;111:775.

21 Santos MS, Gomes JA, Hofling-Lima AL, Rizzo LV, Romano AC, Belfort R Jr: Survival analysis of conjunctival limbal grafts and amniotic membrane transplantation in eyes with total limbal stem cell deficiency. Am J Ophthalmol 2005;140:223.

22 Gillette TE, Chandler JW, Greiner JV: Langerhans cells of the ocular surface. Ophthalmology 1982;89:700.

23 Daya SM, Ilari FA: Living related conjunctival limbal allograft for the treatment of stem cell deficiency. Ophthalmology 2001;108:126.

24 Pellegrini G, Traverso CE, Franzi AT, Zingirian M, Cancedda R, De Luca M: Long-term restoration of damaged corneal surfaces with autologous cultivated corneal epithelium. Lancet 1997;349:990.

25 Meller D, Pires RT, Tseng SC: Ex vivo preservation and expansion of human limbal epithelial stem cells on amniotic membrane cultures. Br J Ophthalmol 2002;86:463.

26 Schwab IR, Reyes M, Isseroff RR: Successful transplantation of bioengineered tissue replacements in patients with ocular surface disease. Cornea 2000;19:421.

27 Tsai RJ, Li LM, Chen JK: Reconstruction of damaged corneas by transplantation of autologous limbal epithelial cells. N Engl J Med 2000;343:86.

28 Koizumi N, Inatomi T, Suzuki T, Sotozono C, Kinoshita S: Cultivated corneal epithelial stem cell transplantation in ocular surface disorders. Ophthalmology 2001;108:1569.

29 Puangsricharern V, Tseng SC: Cytologic evidence of corneal diseases with limbal stem cell deficiency. Ophthalmology 1995;102:1476.

30 Tseng SC, Prabhasawat P, Lee SH: Amniotic membrane transplantation for conjunctival surface reconstruction. Am J Ophthalmol 1997;124:765.

31 Pauklin M, Kakkassery V, Steuhl KP, Meller D: Expression of membrane-associated mucins in limbal stem cell deficiency and after transplantation of cultivated limbal epithelium. Curr Eye Res 2009;34:221.

32 Pauklin M, Steuhl KP, Meller D: Characterization of the corneal surface in limbal stem cell deficiency and after transplantation of cultivated limbal epithelium. Ophthalmology 2009;116:1048.

33 Meller D, Tseng SC: Conjunctival epithelial cell differentiation on amniotic membrane. Invest Ophthalmol Vis Sci 1999;40:878.

34 Koizumi N, Fullwood NJ, Bairaktaris G, Inatomi T, Kinoshita S, Quantock AJ: Cultivation of corneal epithelial cells on intact and denuded human amniotic membrane. Invest Ophthalmol Vis Sci 2000;41:2506.

35 Fuchsluger T, Tuerkeli E, Westekemper H, Esser J, Steuhl KP, Meller D: Rate of epithelialisation and reoperations in corneal ulcers treated with amniotic membrane transplantation combined with botulinum toxin-induced ptosis. Graefes Arch Clin Exp Ophthalmol 2007;245:955.

36 Rama P, Bonini S, Lambiase A, et al: Autologous fibrin-cultured limbal stem cells permanently restore the corneal surface of patients with total limbal stem cell deficiency. Transplantation 2001;72:1478.

37 Sangwan VS, Matalia HP, Vemuganti GK, et al: Clinical outcome of autologous cultivated limbal epithelium transplantation. Indian J Ophthalmol 2006;54:29.

38 Lange C, Feltgen N, Junker B, Schulze-Bonsel K, Bach M: Resolving the clinical acuity categories 'hand motion' and 'counting fingers' using the Freiburg Visual Acuity Test (FrACT). Graefes Arch Clin Exp Ophthalmol 2009;247:137.

39 Shimazaki J, Shimmura S, Tsubota K: Donor source affects the outcome of ocular surface reconstruction in chemical or thermal burns of the cornea. Ophthalmology 2004;111:38.

40 Shortt AJ, Secker GA, Rajan MS, et al: Ex Vivo Expansion and Transplantation of Limbal Epithelial Stem Cells. Ophthalmology 2008.

41 Gomes JA, Santos MS, Ventura AS, Donato WB, Cunha MC, Hofling-Lima AL: Amniotic membrane with living related corneal limbal/conjunctival allograft for ocular surface reconstruction in Stevens-Johnson syndrome. Arch Ophthalmol 2003;121:1369.

42 Holland EJ, Djalilian AR, Schwartz GS: Management of aniridic keratopathy with keratolimbal allograft: a limbal stem cell transplantation technique. Ophthalmology 2003;110:125.

43 Meller D, Kruse F: Ex-vivo expansion of cornea stem cells: experimental principles and initial clinical results (in German). Ophthalmologe 2001;98:811.

44 Meller D, Fuchsluger T, Pauklin M, Steuhl KP: Ocular surface reconstruction in graft-versus-host disease with HLA-identical living-related allogeneic cultivated limbal epithelium after hematopoietic stem cell transplantation from the same donor. Cornea 2009;28:233.

45 Nakamura T, Inatomi T, Sotozono C, et al: Transplantation of autologous serum-derived cultivated corneal epithelial equivalents for the treatment of severe ocular surface disease. Ophthalmology 2006;113:1765.

46 Hernandez Galindo EE, Theiss C, Pauklin M, Wettey FR, Steuhl KP, Meller D: Correlation of cell cycle kinetics with p63 expression in human limbal epithelial cells expanded on intact human amniotic membrane. Ophthalmic Res 2009;41:83.

Daniel Meller, MD
Department of Ophthalmology, University of Duisburg-Essen
Hufelandstrasse 55
DE–45122 Essen (Germany)
Tel. +49 201 723 84382, Fax +49 201 723 5645, E-Mail daniel.meller@uk-essen.de

Brewitt H (ed): Research Projects in Dry Eye Syndrome.
Dev Ophthalmol. Basel, Karger, 2010, vol 45, pp 71–82

Laser Scanning Confocal Microscopy for Conjunctival Epithelium Imaging

Clemens Jürgens[a] · Robert Rath[a] · Jürgen Giebel[b] · Frank H.W. Tost[a]

[a]Department of Ophthalmology, University Hospital, and [b]Institute of Anatomy and Cell Biology, Ernst Moritz Arndt University, Greifswald, Germany

Abstract

Background: Conjunctival disorders may adversely affect tear film and promote/induce the development of sicca syndrome (also known as Sjögren's syndrome). The basic diagnostics of sicca syndrome are slit lamp examination and functional tests (such as the Schirmer test, break-up time, or fluorescein/rose bengal staining). However, morphological analysis requires time and effort, both in terms of technical equipment and labor, and the results are not available immediately. In contrast, when using laser scanning confocal microscopy (LSCM), the anatomy and morphology of the conjunctival epithelium may be evaluated in vivo during the clinical examination. **Material and Methods:** We examined the conjunctival epithelium of 23 subjects with healthy eyes using LSCM. We compared intraindividual morphological patterns of normal conjunctival epithelium derived from the Heidelberg Retina Tomograph II – Rostock Cornea Module (HRTII-RCM) with those from impression cytology. All examinations were performed on the conjunctiva bulbi at the 12 o'clock position, 2 mm from the limbus corneae. **Results:** LSCM and impression cytology examine the conjunctival epithelium from identical perspectives. This facilitates an intraindividual comparison of morphological patterns. In addition, artifact detection and the mapping of light/dark pattern recognition of the LSCM to the microscopy of the impression cytology were reliable. LSCM allows in vivo discrimination of non-secretory from secretory cells in conjunctival epithelium. Non-secretory epithelium shows dark, light and bright cytoplasm of epithelial cells on LSCM, in contrast to impression cytology. Nucleoplasmic ratio ranged from 1:1 to 1:4. Shape, size and interior structure were reliable criteria to distinguish goblet cells from non-secretory cells. The interior structure of the goblet cells showed dark or highly reflective bright homogeneous textures. **Conclusion:** LSCM is a feasible method for examining the morphology of conjunctival epithelium using non-invasive in vivo imaging. Morphological criteria for squamous metaplasia of the conjunctiva in sicca syndrome are already known from cytology, and can be used in almost the same manner in LSCM. The separation of epithelial microcysts from small goblet cells is difficult with LSCM. Finally, the clinical application of LSCM in the staging of sicca syndrome has to be evaluated in future studies.

The conjunctiva is an important part of the epithelial barrier of the ocular surface and is essential to the transparency of the cornea. The mucosal barrier consists of

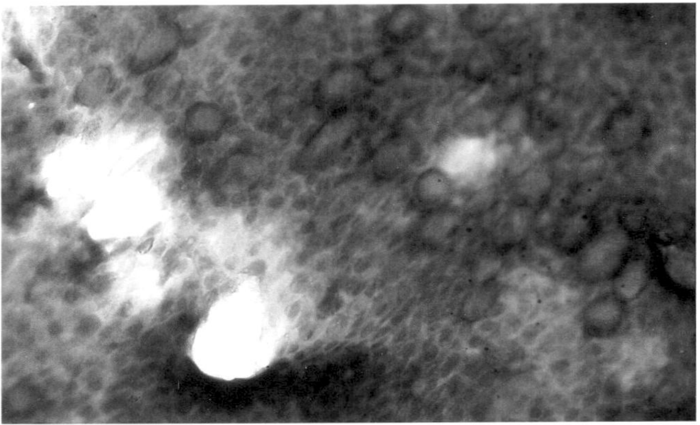

Fig. 1. Impression cytology: normal conjunctival epithelium. Uniform field of non-secretory epithelial cells, nucleoplasmic ratio from 1:1 to 1:2, intermediate PAS-positive goblet cells (light microscopy). PAS-hematoxylin. ×20.

non-keratinizing squamous epithelium with a secretory function (fig. 1) and eye-associated lymphoid tissue.

Numerous non-secretory epithelial cells as well as secretory cells, i.e. goblet cells, can be found in various frequencies. Using extensive transmission electron microscopy, the cellular and molecular structure of conjunctival epithelial cells varies depending on the topographic region. Five different non-secretory epithelial cells as well as epithelial cells with dark, light and bright cytoplasm are currently known [1].

Conjunctival dysfunction affects the tear film, and may promote significant dryness of the ocular surface. Diagnosing sicca syndrome (also known as Sjögren's syndrome) is complicated by the range of symptoms a patient may manifest. Symptoms from sicca syndrome are often similar to those caused by other conditions. Frequently, sicca syndrome causes associated blepharoconjunctivitis, and as a result it is not easy to distinguish whether primary blepharoconjunctivitis or sicca syndrome is the cause of the inflammation. Both diseases have different mechanisms which activate inflammatory responses of varying intensities in the conjunctival epithelium. Just like other chronic diseases, an unnoticed onset together with a slow progression make a reliable diagnosis difficult in sicca syndrome. The ophthalmologist has to treat patients with severe sicca syndrome, as well as patients with mild symptoms or subclinical signs. The latter describes a clinical condition that has been already established in other chronic diseases, e.g. hypertension where drug therapy was adapted to pre-hypertensive conditions. By contrast, in cases of subclinical Sicca syndrome, it is difficult for ophthalmologists to correlate patient-reported symptoms with objective evidence.

All of this illustrates why a combination of several tests is needed for diagnosing and staging sicca syndrome. Testing lacrimal function is easy to perform with the Schirmer test, break-up time, lacrimal osmolarity or fluorescein staining. Morphological imaging is only recommended for staging: Cytobrush, impression cytology or biopsy (guidelines of the Berufsverband der Augenärzte Deutschlands and Deutsche Ophthalmologische Gesellschaft). All of these methods require a minimally invasive or invasive tissue sample with complex sample processing. Consequently, the results are only available after a time delay. Laser scanning confocal microscopy (LSCM) may be a promising technique for non-invasive imaging to determine the in vivo clinical diagnosis of sicca syndrome, especially if comparative patterns of other clinical examinations are available. In this study, we analyzed intraindividual morphological characteristics of human conjunctival epithelium in healthy eyes, comparing assignable and reproducible patterns of LSCM (Heidelberg Retina Tomograph II – Rostock Cornea Module; HRTII-RCM) alongside impression cytology of the conjunctiva.

Materials and Methods

Healthy eyes of 23 subjects were examined using the new in vivo imaging LSCM. A comparative intraindividual structure and pattern recognition was performed in a standardized procedure. Using the HRTII-RCM, a predefined region of the conjunctiva bulbi was examined with a contact method. For reasons of accessibility, we examined the superior conjunctiva bulbi with the in vivo LSCM after the application of local anesthetics (Proparakain®-POS 0.5% proxymetacaine-HCL eye drops). The upper eyelid was retained while the subject looked down. Then the device was attached to the surface of the eye using a contact gel (Vidisic eye gel). This procedure allowed an in vivo examination of the conjunctiva bulbi at the 12 o'clock position, 2–3 mm from the limbus corneae in all 23 subjects.

Following LSCM, and after repeated topical anesthesia with Proparakain®-POS 0.5% eye drops, we took impression cytology specimens from the identical region of the conjunctiva bulbi. In addition, we performed topographic impression cytology of the conjunctiva, and took more cytological samples for microscopy from different regions of the bulbar conjunctiva at 9, 3 and 6 o'clock positions. Each specimen was sampled with a standardized pressure of 50 cN using cellulose acetate membrane filters (Millipore™). The sampled conjunctival epithelium was preserved with a fixing spray and stained with PAS-hematoxylin for light microscopy. Impression cytology is appropriate for comparative pattern recognition because it gives a similar perspective of the sample as in vivo LSCM. Instrument engineering and device handling have been explained in detail in other papers [2, 3].

Results

Table 1 provides an overview of the cellular structures in the conjunctival epithelium in the context of comparing impression cytology to LSCM.

A prerequisite for a reliable intraindividual analysis of morphological differences in conjunctival epithelium derived from established impression cytology compared to the innovative LSCM is a similar anatomical and morphological perspective of the specimen. Both LSCM and impression cytology provide identical perspectives in comparison to conventional histomorphological preparation following surgical excision of the conjunctiva. Consequently, a planar surface of the specimen can be examined instead of a transverse section, which is common in conventional histological

Table 1. Overview of cellular structures of the conjunctival epithelium and their associated patterns in light microscopy compared to LSCM

Morphological feature of the conjunctiva	Patterns in impression cytological specimen using light microscopy (PAS-hematoxylin)	Pattern recognition using in vivo LSCM
Mucin	strip-, dot- or point-shaped PAS-positive granules; clustered diffuse distributed red-stained granules	bright diffuse point-shaped reflectors; discriminable from bright nucleus due to irregular boundary
Goblet cells	circular or oval shape; larger than non-secretory epithelial cells; staining of the interior structure varies (secretion); glycoproteins and mucin stained blue and red	rich in contrast, circular or oval shape, varying size; considerably larger than non-secretory epithelial cells; thick hyperreflective cell borders; interior structure with varying light/dark pattern
Epithelial cells, non-secretory		
Nucleus	saturated, dark-blue grained chromatin structure; circular or oval shape; nucleoplasmic ratio 1:1–1:2	bright, circular or oval structures; nucleoplasmic ratio 1:1–1:2; difficult to differentiate from cytoplasm
Cytoplasm	light blue	low-contrast structure; capable of differentiating from high-contrast structures (nucleus, cell border, intercellular space) due to light/dark distribution
Cell membrane	indistinct linear structure	distinctive lines with bright or dark pixels
Intercellular space	specifiable	clearly specifiable

preparations. This makes the identification of similar patterns of the conjunctival epithelium and the detection of artifacts easier. All 23 healthy subjects showed normal cytomorphological findings of the superficial conjunctival epithelium (fig. 1) using impression cytology [4].

The intraindividual comparison of the impression cytology reference (fig. 1–3) and the in vivo examination of the conjunctival epithelium with the HRTII-RCM (fig. 4–8) led to the following results.

Using LSCM, the epithelial barrier of the conjunctiva can be observed directly.

Superficial epithelial cells of the bulbar conjunctiva were characterized as large loosely arranged cells with a hyporeflective nucleus (fig. 4). Intermediate epithelial

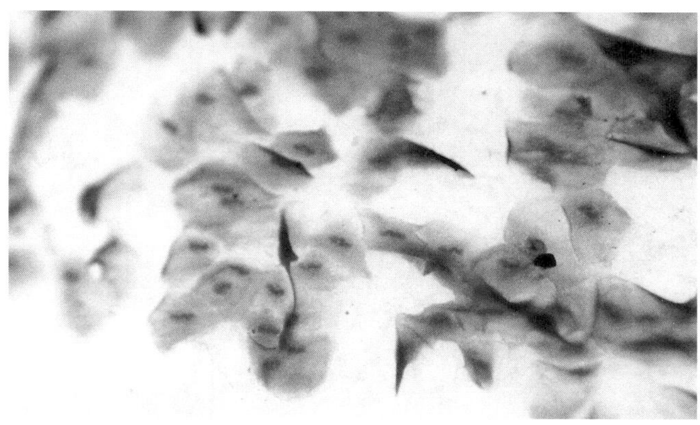

Fig. 2. Squamous metaplasia of the conjunctival epithelium in severely dry eyes. Loose clusters of non-secretory epithelial cells, nucleoplasmic ratio ranges from 1:4 to 1:8, snake-like chromatin; no evidence of goblet cells (impression cytology, light microscopy). PAS-hematoxylin. ×40.

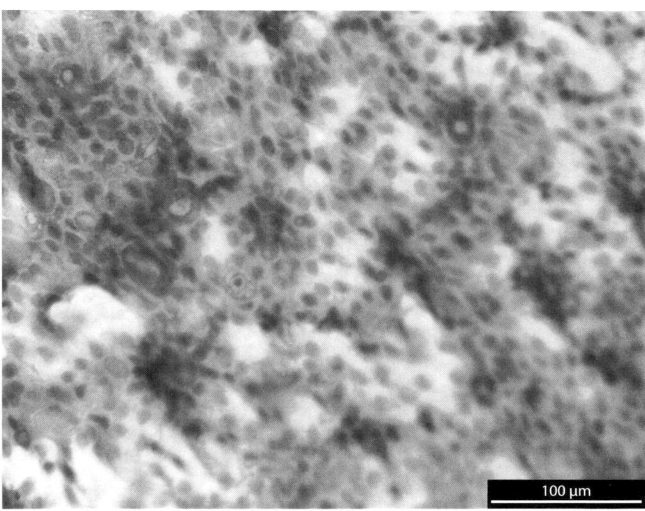

Fig. 3. Impression cytology of the conjunctival epithelium in healthy eyes. The majority of goblet cells appear PAS-positive because they contain glycoprotein and mucin. However, various goblet cells – whose secretion appears to be (partially or totally) unstained – are visible (impression cytology, light microscopy). PAS-hematoxylin. ×20.

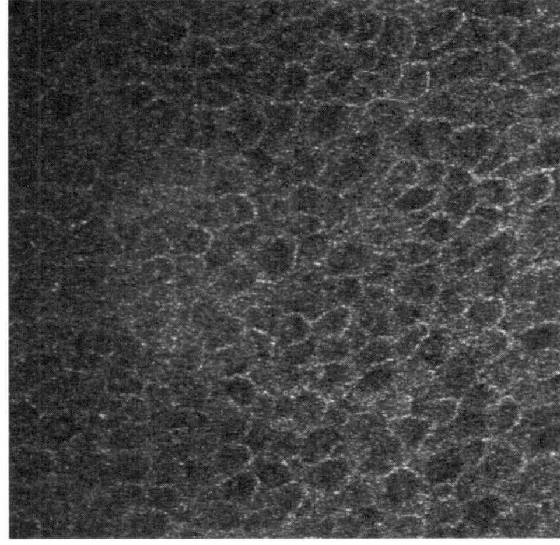

Fig. 4. Uniform field of non-secretory epithelial cells imaged using LSCM. Cell borders and intercellular spaces are observable due to various bright reflections. It is possible to differentiate some of the bright nuclei from the hyporeflective cytoplasm.

Fig. 5. Large goblet cell within a uniform layer of conjunctival epithelial cells imaged using LSCM. The thick cell membrane and the nucleus appear hyperreflective, whereas the cytoplasm is darker.

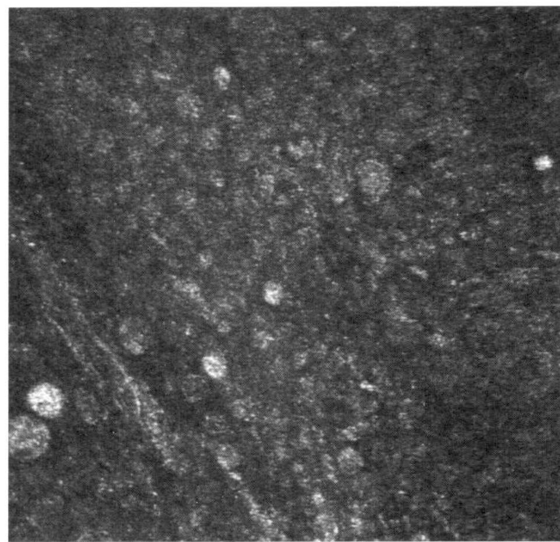

Fig. 6. Several goblet cells in conjunctival epithelium of a healthy subject imaged using LSCM. In contrast to figure 5, the goblet cell lumen is hyperreflective. As a result, the thick cell membrane is not capable of being differentiated.

cells were captured with features of small tightly arranged oval cells with a punctiform hyperreflective nucleus. Basal epithelial cells appeared to be polygonal and arranged regularly within hyperreflective cell borders. The presumed goblet cell was defined as a large hyperreflective oval-shaped cell with relatively homogeneous brightness, crowded in groups or mainly dispersed (fig. 5, 6). The basement membrane, a prominent hyperreflective band, separated epithelial cells from the subepithelial structure. Bulbar conjunctival substantia propria, beneath the basement membrane, was mainly composed of highly vascularized loose connective tissues, which were irregularly arranged fibers or a network of fibers, punctiform hyperreflective immune cells, and sharp tracks of blood vessels.

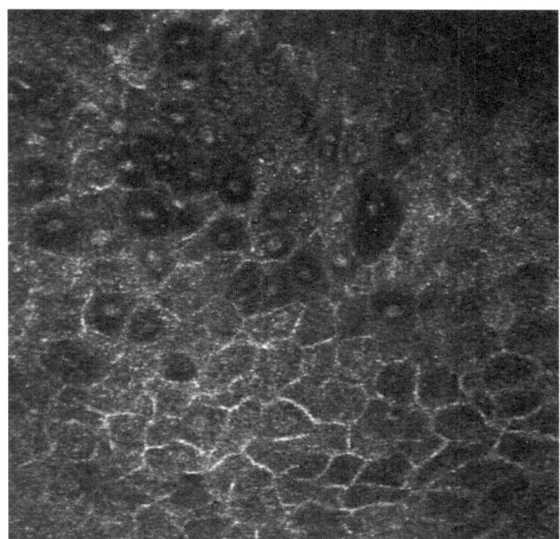

Fig. 7. Uniform layer of non-secretory epithelial cells imaged using LSCM. Just as in transmission electron microscopy, epithelial cells appear bright, dark and intermediate. The cytoplasm shows various bright reflectors. The nucleus can be identified if the cytoplasm is hyporeflective. The nucleoplasmic ratio ranges from 1:2 to 1:4. (in vivo microscopy with LSCM.)

It is possible to differentiate between non-secretory epithelial cells of the conjunctiva bulbi and secretory cells. Polyhexagonal cell borders of non-secretory epithelial cells of stratified non-keratinizing squamous epithelium can be displayed with LSCM. Nucleoplasmic relation can be determined with LSCM in the same way as minimally invasive impression cytology (fig. 7). As expected in all healthy subjects, the nucleoplasmic ratio ranged from 1:1 to 1:2; this did not depend on the imaging method (impression cytology or LSCM) and represents normal findings (fig. 1, 3, 4). Using the morphological in vivo examination, LSCM cell borders appeared hyperreflective, while the cytoplasm showed marginal reflections with dark homogeneous textures. Circular and oval nuclei were rich in contrast and showed various bright reflections. Diffuse punctiform bright reflections between cell groups were a sign of dispersed mucin granuloma. In the superior parts of the superficial conjunctival epithelium, we also found bright linear reflections, which might correspond to crypts of the conjunctival epithelium. Large circular or oval light/dark patterns appeared between the non-secretory epithelial cells. In reference to impression cytology, this light/dark pattern corresponded to the secretory cells of the conjunctival epithelium. The distinction of goblet cells from non-secretory epithelial cells was also possible with the in vivo LSCM on the basis of cell shape, size and interior structure. Goblet cells appeared rich in contrast in cell membranes and the intracellular space with various bright reflections in contrast to the more frequent non-secretory epithelial cells of the conjunctiva. The lumen of the goblet cells was either hyporeflective with various dark reflections (fig. 5) or hyperreflective (fig. 6). In cases of a high reflective interior structure, it was not always possible to differentiate the thicker cell border of secretory goblet cells from the interior structure of the goblet cells using LSCM (fig. 8).

In impression cytology, the interior structure of the non-secretory epithelial cells always appeared in bluish regular coloring. Using in vivo imaging with LSCM, we

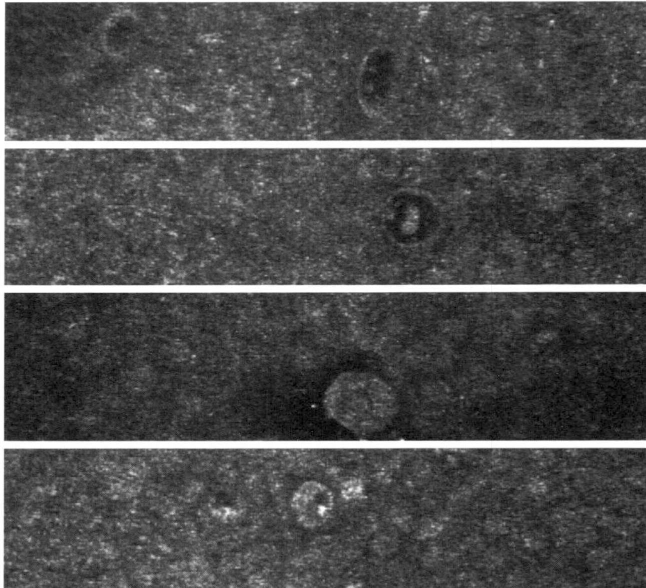

Fig. 8. Using LSCM, goblet cells of the conjunctival epithelium appear with varying reflectivity, in the same manner as in impression cytology.

found corresponding regular low-contrast dark patterns. In addition, we observed groups of non-secretory conjunctival epithelial cells with irregular cytoplasmic light/dark patterns. This morphological characteristic of the conjunctival epithelium is not common for impression cytology, but for transmission electron microscopy (where cytoplasm alternates in dark low-contrast structures), while other epithelial cells of the surrounding area have regular cytoplasmic reflections with various bright intensities. In contrast to impression cytology with LSCM, we were able to differentiate non-secretory epithelial cells with mild dark cytoplasmic reflections from intermediate reflective cytoplasm and bright highly reflective cytoplasmic structures (fig. 1, 7). A similar pattern of the interior structure of the non-secretory conjunctival epithelium was only known from experimental examinations with the transmission electron microscope. However, this method is not feasible for clinical imaging and furthermore requires surgical excision procedures.

Discussion

LSCM together with the HRTII-RCM is a feasible method of analyzing the morphology of the conjunctival epithelial barrier. While clinical examination and quantitative HRT analysis of the optic disc are state-of-the-art in glaucoma monitoring, and retinal examination is the established way to quantify macular edema, we still have to wait for application scenarios for LSCM in vivo examination of the conjunctiva. A fundamental prerequisite for this objective is a systematic analysis of all patterns of healthy conjunctival epithelium. Various research groups have already published first results; however, these only included very few subjects. In 2004, Kobayashi et al. [5] examined initially non-fixed conjunctiva of rabbits. In 2005, the first morphological in vivo results from using the LSCM in 4 healthy volunteers followed. Different parts of the conjunctiva (conjunctiva bulbi, conjunctiva tarsalis et palpebrae) were observed and documented. The cell size of non-secretory epithelial cells varied in relation to the examined region. The conjunctiva tarsalis et palpebrae presented smaller and tighter non-secretory epithelial cells using in vivo LSCM compared to the conjunctiva bulbi. This represents a fact that is already known from topographic impression cytology and ophthalmopathology. In LSCM, we can detect small crypts and conjunctival folding, which is impossible with fixed specimens in impression cytology and histology. Kobayashi et al. [5, 6] even found subepithelial structures of small vessels and demonstrated Langerhans cells with characteristic dendritic patterns. Secretory cells were classified by size and either a circular or oval shape. All goblet cells appeared in a homogeneous structure with various bright reflections. In our studies, we also found goblet cells as described by Kobayashi et al. [5, 6]. Furthermore, we detected secretory cells with a dark interior structure. The thick cell membrane and the intercellular space provide a sharp contrast to the non-secretory epithelial cells. The alternating light/dark pattern of the secretory goblet cells may indicate variations in secretory consistency. Variations in goblet cell secretion are already known from light microscopy with various stainings and the application of histochemistry. On the other hand, this could be a result of different functional conditions of the secretory goblet cells, i.e. hyposecretion following secretory activity. At present, it is difficult to differentiate between microcysts and closed goblet cells. Several reports about detected microcysts have been published [7–9]. Ciancaglini et al. [7] suggested that microcysts of the conjunctival epithelium are pathognomonic for the development of ocular hypertension and glaucoma; however, this hypothesis was disproved in the studies of Efron et al. [8] and Messmer et al. [9]. Microcysts are commonly detected in the conjunctival epithelium of healthy eyes, but their frequency depends on the topography. Microcysts were most frequent in the palpebral conjunctiva, while they were rare in the conjunctiva bulbi of healthy subjects [8, 9]. In contrast to Efron et al. [8], we examined the conjunctiva closer to the limbus corneae. Messmer et al. [9] identified patterns of microcysts in LSCM as closed goblet cells. However, they found a high percentage of patterns in upper epithelial layers which corresponded to oval pyknotic nuclei. From impression cytology, we already know snake-like chromatin, which appears frequently in sicca syndrome, characterizes metaplasia of the conjunctiva. Hence, the authors assumed a subclinical sicca syndrome in all healthy subjects examined. Functional tests to exclude sicca syndrome were not performed in that study [9]. Our results, together with the conclusions of other studies [10–22], provide evidence that LSCM is capable of detecting all important morphological criteria of metaplasia of the conjunctival epithelium in sicca syndrome. Future research with large-scale in vivo examinations of the LSCM is still mandatory. This requirement is supported by the fact that (in contrast to our in vivo examinations of non-secretory conjunctival epithelium with dark, intermediate and bright cytoplasmic structure published in 2006 [15]) Kobayashi did not report similar results of LSCM examinations [5, 6]. In the meantime, other publications have confirmed our observation [8, 9]. Furthermore, in vivo cell counting of the conjunctival epithelium was performed with the HRT3/RCM software [8]. Efron et al. [8] examined the bulbar conjunctiva at the 12 o'clock position, 2–4 mm behind the limbus corneae (mean thickness: 32.9 ± 1.1 μm; overall goblet cell density: 111 ± 58 cells/mm^2), and failed to observe any dendritic Langerhans cells in this part of the conjunctiva, whilst finding 23 ± 25 cells/mm^2 in other topographic regions of the conjunctiva bulbi.

The fundamental advantage of morphological in vivo diagnosis with LSCM is the contemporary non-invasive imaging analysis of the conjunctival epithelial barrier. The results can be interpreted while the patient is present, similarly to various other functional tests for sicca syndrome. So far, diagnostic imaging – such as Cytobrush, impression cytology or even histopathological examination following surgical excision – was only recommended for extended staging of sicca syndrome or chronic conjunctivitis. LSCM could advance to a secondary imaging method for diagnosing disorders of the ocular surface next to the established slit lamp biomicroscopy. Structural cellular imaging would expand the capacity of slit lamp biomicroscopy. Limitations of LSCM are the considerable initial costs and the operating expenses. Examination with the HRTII-RCM requires direct and air-free contact with the surface of the patient's eye. Irregular uneven regions of the eye surface make it difficult to keep the contact free from air and complicate in vivo examination of the palpebral angle or the lacrimal gland. Combined with the HRTII, the accessibility of the conjunctiva is complicated, especially in cases of head immobility, spinal stiffness or postural deformity. Patients with tremor or patients who do not cooperate cannot be examined. Continuous imaging in z-scan mode of all epithelial layers of the conjunctiva and subepithelial connective tissue requires patience on the part of the examiner and a highly cooperative subject. Slight eye movements can cause interfering artifacts. The examination requires direct contact with the conjunctiva, and therefore carries an inherent risk of infection. Due to poor accessibility of the palpebral angle or the lacrimal gland for in vivo examination, these regions require established imaging techniques, such as minimally invasive cytology or histological examination. For major parts of the conjunctiva bulbi and the conjunctiva tarsi, LSCM will become more important for in vivo diagnosis. Several case reports have been published detailing various pathological conditions of the conjunctiva: conjunctival lymphoma, conjunctival amyloidosis, atopic keratoconjunctivitis, pterygium, and pigmented conjunctival tumors [16].

In vivo examination of the conjunctival epithelial barrier will become increasingly important in various disorders of the ocular surface, and especially sicca syndrome. Besides the differentiation of non-secretory epithelial cells and secretory goblet cells, several light/dark patterns – which are based on different functional conditions or the specific molecular morphology of individual cells – are discriminable. Further research is required to compare and analyze differences in pattern recognition of established imaging (i.e. cytology or histopathology) and innovative non-invasive LSCM.

Conclusions

- LSCM is a non-invasive in vivo imaging technique that is capable of analyzing the morphology of the conjunctival epithelium.
- The HRTII-RCM system presents the conjunctival epithelium in a clinical perspective similar to the specimen of impression cytology.
- The LSCM not only allows the examination of superior epithelial cell layers, but also the complete thickness of the conjunctival epithelium.
- It is possible to inspect the morphology of non-secretory and secretory cells in the conjunctival epithelium with LSCM.
- Shape, size and border of goblet cells can be characterized with light/dark patterns of LSCM.
- It is difficult to differentiate epithelial microcysts from small goblet cells using LSCM.
- In LSCM, conjunctival goblet cells have 2 appearances.
- In LSCM, non-secretory epithelial cells are crowded into groups, just as in impression cytological specimen. Small linear hyperreflective structures correspond to crypts and conjunctival folding, which cannot be observed in fixed specimens of impression cytology.
- In LSCM, the cytoplasm of non-secretory epithelial cells shows a homogeneous pattern that is similar to light microscopy. Epithelial cells can be classified into dark, intermediate and bright reflective patterns.
- The nucleoplasmic ratio of conjunctival epithelial cells can be determined in vivo using LSCM.
- With LSCM, the in vivo analysis of the conjunctival epithelial morphology is already possible during the clinical examination.
- Squamous metaplasia of the conjunctival epithelium can be examined with the non-invasive LSCM.
- LSCM can be helpful in diagnosing and staging of the sicca syndrome because relevant morphological criteria of conjunctival metaplasia can be evaluated (goblet cells, transformation of nucleoplasmic ratio, 'snake' cells [11]).
- The clinical value of LSCM in sicca syndrome staging has to be evaluated in future experimental studies.
- Using LSCM, functional lacrimal tests (like the Schirmer test, break-up time and slit lamp biomicroscopy) can be extended yielding important anatomical/morphological information.

References

1 Steuhl KP: Ultrastructure of the conjunctival epithelium. Dev Ophthalmol 1989;19:1–104.

2 Stave J, Zinser G, Grummer G, Guthoff R: Modified Heidelberg Retinal Tomograph HRT: initial results of in vivo presentation of corneal structures. Ophthalmologe 2002;99:276–280.

3 Zhivov A, Beck R, Guthoff R: Corneal and conjunctival findings after mitomycin C application in pterygium surgery: an in vivo confocal microscopy study. Acta Ophthalmol 2009;87:166–172.

4 Tost F: Practical conjunctival cytology. Ophthalmologe 1999;96:276–289.

5 Kobayashi A, Yoshita T, Sugiyama K: In vivo laser and white-light confocal microscopic findings of human conjunctiva. Ophthalmic Surg Lasers Imaging 2004;35:482–484.

6 Kobayashi A, Yoshita T, Sugiyama K: In vivo findings of the bulbar/palpebral conjunctiva and presumed meibomian glands by laser scanning confocal microscopy. Cornea 2005;24:985–988.

7 Ciancaglini M, Carpineto P, Agnifili L, Nubile M, Fasanella V, Mastropasqua L: Conjunctival modifications in ocular hypertension and primary open angle glaucoma: an in vivo confocal microscopy study. Invest Ophthalmol Vis Sci 2008;49:3042–3048.

8 Efron N, Al-Dossari M, Pritchard N: In vivo confocal microscopy of the bulbar conjunctiva. Clin Experiment Ophthalmol 2009;37:335–344.

9 Messmer EM, Mackert MJ, Zapp DM, Kampik A: In vivo confocal microscopy of normal conjunctiva and conjunctivitis. Cornea 2006;25:781–788.

10 Wells AP, Wakely L, Birchall W, Delaney PM: In vivo fibreoptic confocal imaging (FOCI) of the human ocular surface. J Anat 2006;208:197–203.

11 Marner K: 'Snake-like' appearance of nuclear chromatin in conjunctival epithelial cells from patients with keratoconjunctivitis sicca. Acta Ophthalmol 1980;58:849–853.

12 Labbé A, Dupas B, Hamard P, Baudouin C: In vivo confocal microscopy study of blebs after filtering surgery. Ophthalmology 2005;112:1979.

13 Messmer EM, Zapp DM, Mackert MJ, Thiel M, Kampik A: In vivo confocal microscopy of filtering blebs after trabeculectomy. Arch Ophthalmol 2006; 124:1095–1103.

14 Mastropasqua L, Nubile M, Lanzini M, Carpineto P, Toto L, Ciancaglini M: Corneal and conjunctival manifestations in Fabry disease: in vivo confocal microscopy study. Am J Ophthalmol 2006;141:709–718.

15 Rath R, Stave J, Guthoff R, Giebel J, Tost F: In vivo imaging of the conjunctival epithelium using confocal laser scanning microscopy. Ophthalmologe 2006;103: 401–405.

16 Messmer EM, Mackert MJ, Zapp DM, Kampik A: In vivo confocal microscopy of pigmented conjunctival tumors. Graefe's Arch Clin Exp Ophthalmol 2006; 244:1437–1445.

17 Massig JH: Real-time confocal laser scan microscope for the examination and diagnosis of the eye in vivo. Appl Opt 1994;33:690–694.

18 Zapp DM, Mackert MJ, Kampik A, Messmer EM: In vivo confocal microscopy of normal conjunctiva and conjunctivitis. Invest Ophthalmol Vis Sci 2005; 46(E-abstract):2732.

19 Bozkurt B, Kiratli H, Soylemezoglu F, Irkec M: In vivo confocal microscopy in a patient with conjunctival amyloidosis. Clin Experiment Ophthalmol 2008; 36:173–175.

20 Pichierri P, Martone Gianluca, Loffredo A, Traversi C, Polito E: In vivo confocal microscopy in a patient with conjunctival lymphoma. Clin Experiment Ophthalmol 2008;36:67–69.

21 Hu Y, Sato Adan E, Matsumoto Y, Dogru M, Fukagawa K, Takano Y, Tsubota K, Fujishima H: Conjunctival in vivo confocal scanning laser microscopy in patients with atopic keratoconjunctivitis. Mol Vis 2007;13:1379–1389.

22 Dhaliwal JS, Kaufman SC, Chiou AG: Current applications of clinical confocal microscopy. Curr Opin Ophthalmol 2007;18:300–307.

Prof. Dr. Frank Tost
Klinik und Poliklinik für Augenheilkunde, Ernst-Moritz-Arndt-Universität Greifswald
Ferdinand-Sauerbruch-Strasse
DE–17475 Greifswald (Germany)
Tel. +49 3834 865 923, Fax +49 3834 865 950, E-Mail tost@uni-greifswald.de

Brewitt H (ed): Research Projects in Dry Eye Syndrome.
Dev Ophthalmol. Basel, Karger, 2010, vol 45, pp 83–92

Pollen Enzymes Degrade Human Tear Fluid and Conjunctival Cells: An Approach to Understanding Seasonal Non-Allergic Conjunctivitis

Dieter Franz Rabensteiner · Eva Spreitzhofer · Gabriele Trummer · Christine Wachswender · Sieglinde Kirchengast · Jutta Horwath-Winter · Otto Schmut

Department of Ophthalmology, Medical University of Graz, Graz, Austria

Abstract

Background: During pollen seasons, allergy-like symptoms can be observed in proven non-allergy sufferers. Pollen enzymes are thought to be responsible for conjunctival irritation. We investigated the influence of the well-known aggressive pollen species hazelnut (*Corylus avellana*) and birch pollen (*Betula pendula*) on both human tear fluid and conjunctival cell cultures. This study is an approach to seasonal non-allergic conjunctivitis (SNAC) syndrome. **Methods:** Zymography was carried out in order to investigate the proteolytic activity of the pollen. Thereafter, human tear fluid was incubated with pollen extract, and the results were studied by polyacrylamide gel electrophoresis. In addition, cultivated conjunctival cells (CHANG cells) were incubated with pollen extracts. Cytomorphological changes were analyzed using the CASY1 Cell Counter. Cell viability was quantified via MTS assay. The viability of the cells which were incubated with pollen extract was compared to the viability of control cells. **Results:** Pollen proteases destroy tear fluid proteins, as observed by polyacrylamide gel electrophoresis. The treatment of CHANG cells with pollen extract induced a statistically significant decrease in cell viability, depending on the pollen extract concentration and the incubation period. **Conclusion:** Evidence of the destruction of tear fluid proteins and damage to human conjunctival cells by pollen proteases explains conjunctival irritation in proven non-allergic people during the pollen season. One reason why not all people are affected by SNAC syndrome to the same extent could be differences in the concentrations of antiproteases present on the ocular surface.

During pollen season, many people suffer from red, watery, itchy and/or sticky eyes, as well as a runny nose, and these symptoms are being observed among proven non-allergy sufferers more frequently. This disease was recently described as seasonal non-allergic conjunctivitis (SNAC) syndrome [1–3].

Our study makes a contribution to the understanding of in vivo reactions in pollen-exposed eyes suffering from SNAC syndrome. We investigated the influence of hazelnut and birch pollen extracts on human tear fluid and conjunctival cells.

Even dry eye symptoms can be caused by pollen [3, 4]. As allergies have increased over the last couple of years, a rising number of patients have been seen in the Department of Ophthalmology, Medical University Graz, Austria, who were found to be suffering from dry eyes due to allergic reactions to various substances. However, a connection between the SNAC syndrome and dry eyes may also exist.

Methods

Pollen Collection

The experiments were carried out with well-known aggressive pollen species, i.e. hazelnut (*Corylus avellana*) and birch pollen (*Betula pendula*). Male inflorescences, which contain pollen, were collected from trees in the local area. Afterwards, they were dried, sieved and stored in paper bags at room temperature.

Zymography

Zymography was performed to investigate the proteolytic activity of pollen with a 10% zymogram gelatin gel, and staining was carried out using a colloidal blue staining kit (both from Invitrogen Life Technologies, Carlsbad, Calif., USA).

Hazelnut pollen (10 mg) and birch pollen (10 mg), which were used in comparison, were incubated with 100 µl physiological saline for 1 h at room temperature. The next day, the pollen extract was centrifuged at 10,000 rpm for 5 min. Then, 15 µl of the supernatant was diluted with sample buffer at a ratio of 1:1. The remaining extract was filtered sterilely, and again 15 µl was diluted with the sample buffer at a ratio of 1:1. Next, 20 µl of the samples were added to each well, and the gel was placed in an electrophoresis chamber filled with running buffer. Zymography was performed for 60 min at 125 V.

Afterwards, the zymogram gel was fixed with renaturing buffer for 30 min at room temperature and developed in developing buffer overnight at 37°C.

The gel was stained with colloidal blue and destained with distilled water. The zymographic spectra were documented by a Minolta RD-175 digital camera.

Collection of Tear Fluid

Tear fluid (25 µl) was collected from healthy test participants with normal tear function after they gave informed consent. Tears were collected from the lower lateral tear meniscus with a capillary tube after stimulation with China mint oil applied to the skin in the area of the zygomatic bone. The samples were transferred into plastic microtubes (Brand GmbH, Wertheim, Germany) and used for the experiment.

Polyacrylamide Gel Electrophoresis

Physiological saline (100 µl) and tear fluid (100 µl), respectively, were laced with 10 mg pollen and incubated at 37°C for 1 h. Afterwards, the mixture was centrifuged at 10,000 rpm for 5 min. Subsequently, 30 µl pollen extract, 5 µl pollen-tear fluid mixture and 5 µl tear fluid, respectively, were diluted with NuPAGE LDS 4× sample buffer at a ratio of 3:1. Pollen extract (15 µl), pollen-tear fluid mixture (4 µl) and pure tear fluid (4 µl), respectively, were pipetted into the wells of the precast NuPAGE 4–12% Bis-Tris gel, 1.0 mm × 10 wells (Invitrogen Life Technologies). Electrophoresis was performed at 200 V and 78 mA for 35 min, after which the gels were fixed in water-methanol-acetic acid (5:6:1) for 10 min, stained overnight with a colloidal blue stain kit (Invitrogen Life Technologies) and destained with distilled water. The electrophoresis patterns were documented by a Minolta RD-175 digital camera.

Pollen Extract for Experiments with CHANG Cells

Dulbecco's modified Eagle medium (DMEM; 12 ml; Invitrogen) and 1% P/S (penicillin/streptomycin, Biochrom, Berlin, Germany) were added to 60 mg and 300 mg of birch pollen, respectively, which equals a concentration of 5 mg and 25 mg birch pollen per ml medium. The pollen suspension was incubated for 24 h at 4°C. Finally, the suspension was centrifuged at 4,500 rpm for 5 min and the supernatant was filtered sterilely to receive the pollen extract needed for the experiments.

Human Conjunctival Cells

Human conjunctival cells (CHANG cells, CCL-20.2, clone 1-5c-4m, Wong-Kilbourne derivates of CHANG conjunctiva) acquired from the American Type Culture Collection (Manassas, Va., USA) were used. This cell line is thought to be derived from normal epithelial conjunctiva, and is immortalized with HeLa marker chromosomes. The cells are positive for keratin and they grow adherently.

The cells were frozen at –196°C in fluid nitrogen. Before use, they were defrosted and resuspended in 10 ml culture medium. To remove dimethyl sulfoxide, they were centrifuged at 800 rpm for 5 min, resuspended in 1,000 μl culture medium and transferred into a 25-cm^2 culture flask purchased from Sarstedt GmbH (Wiener Neudorf, Austria). Finally, 4 ml DMEM containing 1% P/S and 10% fetal bovine serum (PAA Laboratories, Pasching, Austria) were added to the flask and incubated in a CO_2 incubator (Heracell 240, Kendro Heraeus, Berlin, Germany) at 37°C. Every 2–3 days, the medium was changed.

The assessment of cell growth, degree of confluence and photo documentation were performed by an inverse microscope (Axio Observer Z.1, Zeiss, Germany). As soon as the cells were at least 90% confluent, they were used for the experiments.

Cell Suspension

Firstly, cell culture medium was removed and the cells were rinsed with rinsing solution (Dulbecco's phosphate buffered saline, DPBS; Invitrogen). Trypsin (1 ml) was added to the cell monolayer, and the flask was returned to the incubator for 2 min. The detachment of the cells was assessed under the microscope. In order to inactivate the effect of trypsin, the cells were resuspended in 3–5 ml medium. Afterwards, the cell suspension was transferred into a centrifuge tube and centrifuged at 800 rpm for 5 min. Finally, the medium was decanted and the cells were resuspended in 2 ml medium.

To receive a cell suspension with the desired cell density, cell count was determined by the CASY®1 Cell Counter + Analyzer System (model TT; Schärfe System, Reutlingen, Germany).

The CASY1 Cell Counter is used to control the quality of cell cultures. The cells are suspended in isotonic measuring solution (CASYton) and aspirated through a precision capillary with a defined size. While passing through the measuring capillary, they are scanned with a frequency of 10^6 measurements per second in a low-voltage field between 2 platinum electrodes. The resulting electrical signals give information about amount, concentration, diameter, volume and size distribution of the cells.

CASYton (9.9 ml) and cell suspension (100 μl) were pipetted into a CASY cup and placed into the counter. After CASY1 cell amount determination, the cell volume with desired cell density was calculated. Cell suspensions with an empiric cell density of 50,000 cells/ml for CASY1 cell analysis and 30,000 cells/ml for the MTS assay were created.

CASY1 Analysis of Cytomorphological Changes

For analysis of cytomorphological changes in human conjunctival cells after the incubation with pollen extracts, 2-ml cell suspensions (50,000 cells/ml) were seeded into 12-well plates (Becton Dickinson and Company, Franklin Lakes, USA) by a pipette (Eppendorf Research, Hamburg, Deutschland). The outer wells of the plate were filled with distilled water, in order to avoid evaporation.

After incubation time of 24 h at 37°C in the CO_2 incubator, cell growth was assessed by an inverse microscope. Cell culture medium was removed and the cells were rinsed with DMEM plus 1% P/S. Next, 1 ml DMEM plus 1% P/S was filled into the control wells and 1 ml pollen extract, obtained from either 5 mg/ml or 25 mg/ml, was applied to the sample wells. Then the plates were incubated for 5 and 24 h, respectively, at 37°C in a CO_2 incubator.

Subsequently, the plates were taken out of the incubator and cytomorphological changes were assessed by the inverse microscope and photo documented. Cell culture medium was removed, after which the cells were rinsed with DPBS rinsing solution and trypsinized with 200 µl trypsin. Finally, the cell suspension and 9.8 ml CASYton were pipetted into a CASY cup and analyzed by the CASY1 system.

Determination of Cell Viability by MTS Assay

Evaluation of cell viability was performed by the Cell Titer 96® Aqueous One Solution Cell Proliferation Assay (MTS) from Promega (Madison, Wisc., USA). The MTS assay is a colorimetric method for determination of the number of viable cells in proliferation, cytotoxicity or chemosensitivity assays. Yellow tetrazolium salt, MTS (Sigma, Germany), is bioreduced to purple formazan in the mitochondria of metabolically active cells. The reduction only takes place when mitochondrial reductase enzymes are active, and therefore conversion can directly be related to the number of viable cells.

Experiments were performed in 96-well microtiterplates (Becton Dickenson) by applying 200 µl cell suspension with a cell density of 30,000 cells per ml into each well using a multichannel pipette (Eppendorf Research, Hamburg, Deutschland). The outer wells of the plate were filled with distilled water in order to avoid evaporation. After an incubation time of 24 h at 37°C in a CO_2 incubator, cell growth was assessed and pollen extract was applied.

Firstly, medium was removed and each well was rinsed twice with 30 µl DMEM plus 1% P/S. Next, 100 µl DMEM plus 1% P/S were filled into the blank wells and 100 µl pollen extract were applied to blank plus pollen wells and the sample wells; 100 µl DMEM plus 1% P/S were filled into the control wells. Finally, the plates were incubated for 5 and 24 h, respectively, at 37°C in a CO_2 incubator.

After 5 and 24 h, respectively, the 96-well plates were taken out of the incubator and cytomorphological changes were assessed by an inverse microscope and photo documented. Cell medium was removed, each well was rinsed with DMEM plus 1% P/S, and 100 µl fresh DMEM plus 1% P/S were applied. Subsequently, 10 µl MTS reagent was added and the plates were incubated for 2 h at 37°C.

After incubation, the plates were evaluated. The absorbance of the MTS reaction product was measured at wavelengths of 492 and 620 nm using an ELISA reader (Anthos 2010, ADAP software from Anthos Labtec Instruments GmbH, Krefeld, Germany).

Statistical Analysis

We calculated the cell viability (as a percentage) on basis of the MTS assay's extinctions. The extinctions of the control cells of each microtiterplate were defined as 100% cell viability for the particular microtiterplate.

All data were analyzed using SPSS 17 (SPSS Inc. Chicago, Ill., USA). The groups were evaluated for parametric or non-parametric distribution by the Kolmogorov-Smirnov test. The cell viability

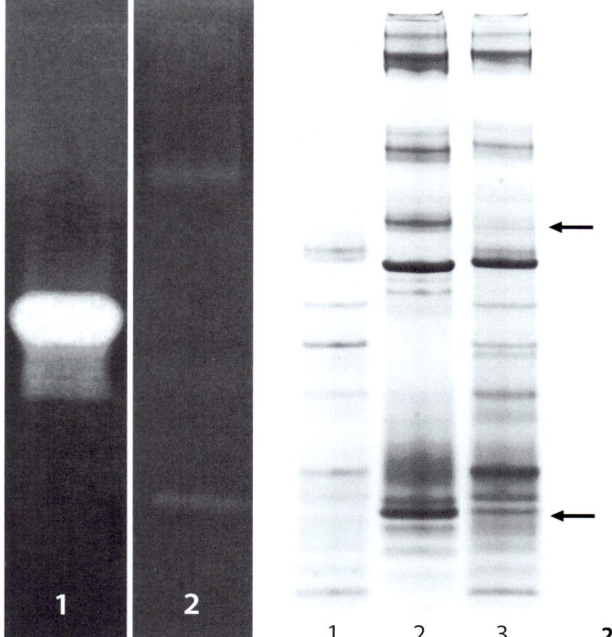

Fig. 1. Zymography pattern of hazelnut (lane 1) and birch pollen extract (lane 2).

Fig. 2. Electrophoresis spectrum of hazelnut pollen extract and tear fluid. Lane 1 = hazelnut pollen; lane 2 = tear fluid; lane 3 = tears incubated with hazelnut pollen extract. After incubation of tear fluid with pollen extract, single bands of the electrophoresis spectrum of tear fluid disappeared (arrows).

of the cells incubated with pollen extract was compared to the control, and evaluated by Mann-Whitney U tests for 2 independent samples. A significance level of $p = 0.05$ and a confidence level of 95% were defined for all statistical analyses.

Results

Zymography

It could be verified that the pollen used for the experiments contains proteases that possess enzymatic activity (fig. 1). The zymographic spectra of the 2 pollen species differed from each other.

Polyacrylamide Gel Electrophoresis

Polyacrylamide gel electrophoresis was performed in order to analyze the proteins of pollen and tear fluid. As an example of the proteolytic activity of pollen, figure 2 shows the electrophoresis spectra of hazelnut pollen extract, tear fluid and tear fluid incubated with pollen extract. Interestingly, after incubation of tear fluid with pollen extract, single bands of the electrophoresis spectrum of tear fluid disappeared. This indicates that some pollen proteins exert proteolytic activity that destroys tear fluid proteins.

Similar results can be obtained using birch pollen extract (not shown).

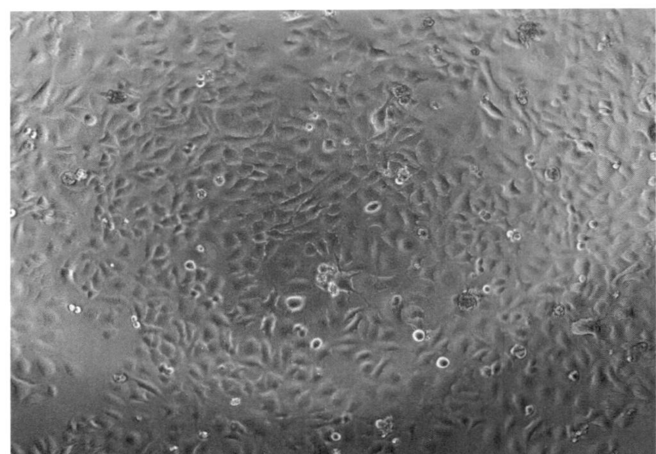

Fig. 3. CHANG cells without pollen addition (control).

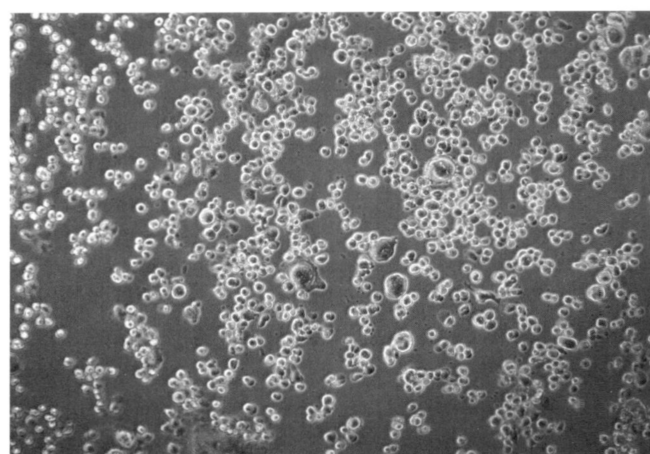

Fig. 4. CHANG cells incubated with birch pollen extract at a concentration of 25 mg/ml after 5 h.

Microscopic Analysis of Cell Cultures Following Incubation with Pollen Extract

Assessment of the cells under the inverse microscope revealed that, compared to the control (fig. 3), cells treated with birch pollen extract showed severe structural changes (fig. 4). Similar results can be obtained with hazelnut pollen extract (not shown).

CASY1 Cell Analysis

Measurements of the cells incubated with pollen extract showed (in comparison to cells without pollen treatment) the cell amount, diameter and volume changed noticeably following incubation with 5 and 25 mg/ml birch pollen extract for incubation times of 5 and 24 h, respectively (table 1). The analysis indicated that the changes

Table 1. CASY1 analysis: cytomorphological changes

Concentration	Incubation time, h	Cell count, %	Cell diameter, %	Cell volume, %
5 mg/ml	0	100.00	100.00	100.00
	5	108.96	99.33	97.54
	24	96.17	99.63	96.74
25 mg/ml	0	100.00	100.00	100.00
	5	72.89	103.06	109.78
	24	17.39	95.70	97.48

were consistent with cell damage. The degree of cell damage depended on the concentration of the pollen extract and incubation time.

MTS Assay

MTS analysis of pollen revealed that pollen possess spontaneous dehydrogenase activity. Therefore, the use of 2 different blanks was necessary to cut out the reagent basic activity and the pollen dehydrogenase activity, respectively. Both blanks were deducted from the corresponding control wells and sample wells.

Incubation of human conjunctival cells with 5 mg birch pollen per ml cell culture medium for 5 h reduced mean cell viability to 88.49%. At an incubation time of 24 h, a reduction to 74.02% cell viability could be observed (fig. 5).

Furthermore, it could be observed that incubation of conjunctival cells with 25 mg birch pollen per ml cell culture medium for 5 h reduced the mean cell viability to 80.49% and for 24 h to 21.96% compared to the control (fig. 5).

Similar results can be obtained with hazelnut pollen extract (not shown).

The extent of the decrease in cell viability depended on the concentration of the pollen extract and incubation time.

The evaluation of our data by the Kolmogorov-Smirnov test showed a non-parametric distribution when evaluating all cells incubated with pollen. The results of the Mann-Whitney U test revealed that the incubation of human conjunctival cells with pollen extract led to a statistically significant decrease in cell viability ($p < 0.000$).

Discussion

Biochemical analysis of pollen has revealed there are numerous different proteins within pollen that vary between the plant species. By performing zymography, some

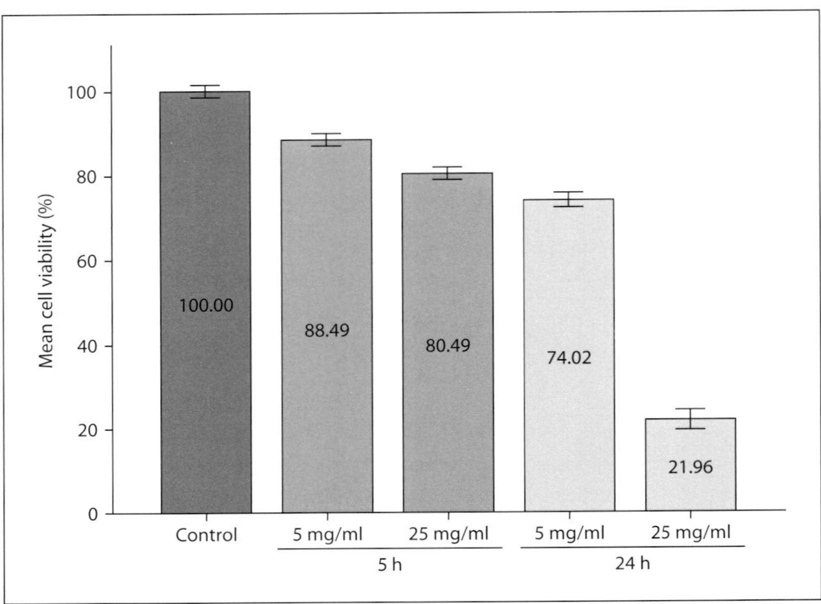

Fig. 5. Mean cell viability of human conjunctival cells after incubation with 5 mg/ml and 25 mg/ml of birch pollen extract for 5 and 24 h, respectively.

of the proteins could be identified as proteases, which were proteolytically active. It could simultaneously be proven that different pollen species contain different types of proteases with varying enzymatic activity [4–8]. These enzymes are of importance in SNAC syndrome [1, 2].

Incubation of dried pollen with any fluid showed that pollen bloat and release their contents, which include proteases, through little pores in the membrane into their surroundings.

This reaction causes the destruction of tear fluid proteins and is thought to destabilize the tear film, which is built through the interaction between proteins, lipids and mucous substances. Tears are no longer able to moisten the affected areas, leading to dry sites on the ocular surface and causing unpleasant irritation [4].

Our experiments showed that treatment of human conjunctival cells with pollen extracts leads to cytomorphological changes consistent with cell damage and to a significant reduction in cell viability. These indicate that exposure of eyes to pollen-polluted surroundings may also lead to conjunctival damage in vivo. Detailed in vivo data on the residence time of pollen on the ocular surface, as observed recently, show that pollen are detectable for up to 5 h on the ocular surface [9], time enough to exert their enzymatic activity.

One reason why not all humans are affected by SNAC syndrome may be differences in the concentration of antiproteases on the ocular surface. Antiproteases and protease inhibitors are contained within body fluids, which usually provide enough protection against proteases. In human tear fluid and nasal secrete, antiproteases such as α_1-antitrypsin, α_1-antichymotrypsin and α_2-macroglobulin can be found [3]. The most important role, as far as quantity is concerned, is played by α_1-antitrypsin. It is an acute phase protein that is able to protect tissues against trypsin and other serine proteases [10, 11]. Therefore, if a sufficient amount of α_1-antitrypsin is present, it is able to inhibit certain pollen proteases.

It can be assumed that when there is a reduction in the quantity or quality of protective factors, proteases can take effect more easily. For example, patients suffering from dry eye syndrome may be more susceptible to protease reactions, as only a reduced amount of antiproteases reach the ocular surface. It seems feasible that a possible accumulation of etiological factors of dry eye, such as exposure to wind, ultraviolet light and ozone, may lead to an increased sensibility to pollen proteases [12–15].

Assessment of cells with the inverse microscope showed that the under normal circumstances adherently growing CHANG cells were detached and floating after treatment with pollen extract. This loss of cell coherence is probably due to a proteolytic degradation of intracellular contact proteins [16]. Experiments with human alveolar epithelial cells incubated with serine endopeptidases of pollen of *Parietaria judaica* showed that not only the pollen extract but also isolated serine proteases led to a loss of cell coherency [17]. This reaction is based on the cleavage of the zonula occludens 1, a cytoplasmatic protein of tight junctions. Destruction of tight junctions enables the invasion of allergens. However, it is still not clear whether pollen proteases are able to destroy tight junctions directly or if the damage is based on an indirect mechanism [17]. It is well known that due to proteolytic damage of tight junctions the epithelial barrier is broken and harmful noxae, like allergens, are able to invade the epithelium, which in turn enables the development of inflammatory or allergic reactions [16].

Allergy as well as non-allergy sufferers can have pollen protease reactions, since the etiological mechanism of the proteolytic pollen reaction is independent of an allergic sensitization. Through our studies, it should be apparent that common treatment options prescribed for allergy sufferers (like H_1-antagonists, cromoglycates and desensitization) are ineffective against proteolytic damage to superficial structures by pollen proteases. An additional deficiency of lacrimal antiproteases may lead to aggravation of the symptoms.

A lot of research has to be done to develop a medication that is actually able to control the protease reaction and its consequences. One approach would be the development of eye drops containing antiproteases or enzyme inhibitors [18]. Unfortunately, the enormous variety of enzymes contained within pollen may complicate this, since most of these proteases have not yet even been specified [19], and also lipases and glycosidases may contribute to the SNAC syndrome. Therefore, specification of these enzymes would be the basis for the development of new treatment options. Until effective medication is established, only common prevention measures to reduce pollen exposure can be recommended.

References

1 Eriksson NE: Seasonal non-allergic rhinoconjunctivitis: a disease caused by pollution? Grana 1991;30: 115–118.

2 Wedback A, Enbom H, Eriksson NE, Moverare R, Malcus I: Seasonal non-allergic rhinitis (SNAR)–a new disease entity? A clinical and immunological comparison between SNAR, seasonal allergic rhinitis and persistent non-allergic rhinitis. Rhinology 2005;43:86–92.

3 Wolf H: Destruction of nasal mucus proteins by pollen proteases; dissertation, Medical University of Graz, 2008.

4 Schmut O, Wolf H, Traunwieser E, Horwath-Winter J: Non-allergic pollen reaction of the eye. Z prakt Augenheilkd 2009;30:139–142.

5 Bagarozzi DA Jr, Pike R, Potempa J, Travis J: Purification and characterization of a novel endopeptidase in ragweed (*Ambrosia artemisiifolia*) pollen. J Biol Chem 1996;271:26227–26232.

6 Matheson NR, Travis J: Purification and characterization of a novel peptidase (IImes) from mesquite (*Prosopis velutina*) pollen. J Biol Chem 1998;273: 16771–16777.

7 Radlowski M: Proteolytic enzymes from generative organs of flowering plants (Angiospermae). J Appl Genet 2005;46:247–257.

8 Raftery MJ, Saldanha RG, Geczy CL, Kumar RK: Mass spectrometric analysis of electrophoretically separated allergens and proteases in grass pollen diffusates. Respir Res 2003;4:10.

9 Rabensteiner DF, Spreitzhofer E, Kirchengast S, Wachswender C, Horwath-Winter J, Schmut O: Die Verweildauer von Pollen an der Augenoberfläche – erste Beobachtungen in-vivo. Spektrum Augenheilkd 2009;23:343–346.

10 Gupta AK, Sarin GS, Mathur MD, Ghosh B: Alpha 1-antitrypsin and serum albumin in tear fluids in acute adenovirus conjunctivitis. Br J Ophthalmol 1988;72:390–393.

11 Talamo RC: Basic and clinical aspects of the alpha1-antitrypsin. Pediatrics 1975;56:91–99.

12 Horwath J, Schmut O: The influence of environmental factors on the development of dry eye. Contactologia 2000;22:21–29.

13 Schmut O, Faulborn J: Zerstörung menschlicher Tränenproteine durch Autoabgase und Zigarettenrauch. Spektrum Augenheilkd 1996;10:176–178.

14 Schmut O, Gruber E, El-Shabrawi Y, Faulborn J: Destruction of human tear proteins by ozone. Free Rad Biol Med 1994;17:165–169.

15 Wedrich A, Schmut O, Rabensteiner DF: Trockenes Auge – Alles zum Sicca-Syndrom. Vienna, Verlagshaus der Ärzte, 2009.

16 Runswick S, Mitchell T, Davies P, Robinson C, Garrod DR: Pollen proteolytic enzymes degrade tight junctions. Respirology 2007;12:834–842.

17 Cunha A: Effect of pollen extract of *Parietaria judaica* in epithelial pulmonary cells. RNA Mensageiro 2003. www1.ci.uc.pt/rnam/artigos/004.htm.

18 Suzuki M, Itoh M, Ohta N, Nakamura Y, Moriyama A, Matsumoto T, Ohashi T, Murakami S: Blocking of protease allergens with inhibitors reduces allergic responses in allergic rhinitis and other allergic diseases. Acta Otolaryngol 2006;126:746–751.

19 Radlowski M, Bartkowiak S, Winiarczyk K, Kalinowski A: Differential influence of bacitracin on plant proteolytic enzyme activities. Biochim Biophys Acta 2005;1722:1–5.

Dr. Dieter Franz Rabensteiner
Department of Ophthalmology, Medical University of Graz
Auenbruggerplatz 4
AT–8036 Graz (Austria)
Tel. +43 316 385 2590, Fax +43 316 385 4159, E-Mail dieter.rabensteiner@medunigraz.at

Brewitt H (ed): Research Projects in Dry Eye Syndrome.
Dev Ophthalmol. Basel, Karger, 2010, vol 45, pp 93–107

Towards a New in vitro Model of Dry Eye: The ex vivo Eye Irritation Test

Felix Spöler[a] · Markus Frentz[b,c] · Norbert F. Schrage[b,c]

[a]Institute of Semiconductor Electronics, RWTH Aachen University, [b]Aachen Center of Technology Transfer in Ophthalmology and [c]Department of Ophthalmology Aachen University, Aachen, Germany

Abstract

Understanding of dry eye syndrome (DES) today is driven by in vivo analysis of tear osmolarity, tear film break up time, impression cytology and description of symptoms. Existing in vivo models of DES need severe alterations of tear production or corneal integrity. For a more detailed analysis of DES under particular environmental and treatment conditions a considerable lack of in vitro methods exists. The main disadvantage of current in vitro models is the limited experimental time frame of only several hours and the impossibility to evaluate healing of epithelial defects. In the present study, evidence is given that these restrictions can be overcome by modifying the established Ex Vivo Eye Irritation Test (EVEIT) to realize a model system for DES. This test is based on abattoir rabbit eyes allowing an experimental time frame of up to 21 days using self-healing corneal cultures. In first experiments it is demonstrated that different severity levels of dry eye can be simulated in the EVEIT system. High-resolution optical coherence tomography (OCT) is applied to monitor the initial phase of DES under evaporative stress acting on the cornea. We observed changes in corneal layer thicknesses and in scattering properties of the stroma, which are sensitive indicators of environmental stress leading to irritation of the ocular surface under dry eye conditions. The combination of corneal culture under desiccating conditions and OCT monitoring offers a new perspective in understanding and treating of DES and is expected to allow for significant pharmacological screening tests.

The integrity of corneal epithelium depends on a constant supply of healthy tears [1]. Dry eye syndrome (DES) is caused by a deficiency in tear production or an inordinate amount of tear evaporation during the open-eye state, leading to an unstable tear film [2]. Tear fluid deficiency results in weakening of the corneal infection barrier and drying up of the superficial corneal epithelium, which subsequent leads to ocular surface damage and increased risk of sight-threatening corneal infection and ulceration [3–5]. DES is associated with a wide spectrum of symptoms, such as itching, grittiness, pain, blurred vision, and in severe cases visual disability or blindness [6, 7], and represents one of the most frequently established diagnoses in ophthalmology

[8]. A number of epidemiological studies have consistently documented a significant increase in the prevalence of DES with age. The incidence is in the range of 10–33% in the population aged more than 65 years, depending on the structure of the study [9–11]. In addition to age-related DES, air conditioning and low humidity have been identified to be the origin of initial symptoms of DES [12]. Recently, a large-scale survey confirmed reduced health-related quality of life in patients with primary Sjögren's syndrome, expressed by (for example) higher hospitalization rates as well as significantly greater depression and cognitive symptoms when compared to a control group [13].

Because of its high incidence, the accompanying limitations in quality of life and its potentially severe consequences, numerous clinical and experimental studies have been conducted to examine the multifactorial immunopathogenesis and develop appropriate treatment strategies for DES [14–18]. Dry eye animal models play an important role in this research and are applied to study pathogenesis, diagnosis and therapy. Here, mainly in vivo models of rabbits, mice, rats, cats, dogs and monkeys have been developed to mimic the multiplicity of pathophysiological mechanisms involved [2, 5, 19, 20]. Live animal models, which are used to examine quantitative tear film deficiency and environmental stress, use surgical removal, irradiation or closure of the lacrimal gland excretory duct [21–23], prevention of eyelid closure [24], drug-induced suppression of tear secretion [5] and increased tear evaporation in a controlled low-humidity environment [25], optionally supplemented by a reduced blinking frequency induced by physical strain [26].

Since corneal inflammation, for example, induces increased lacrimation [27], changes in the tear secretion or goblet cell secretion (as a reaction to the externally forced dry eye conditions) are likely within these models. These unknown parameters can have an evident effect on the significance of the results obtained [4]. In addition, to achieve statistical certainty in spite of interindividual differences, extensive series of animal experiments have to be performed, which are time-consuming and resource-intensive. Therefore, reliable and highly standardized methods are required to provide economic and logistical advantages. One potential avenue is to replace animal tests by organotypic living models in research and pharmacological tests investigating specific problems in dry eye.

Many intrinsic parameters like immune, endocrine and neuronal factors can only be modeled using living organisms. In contrast, investigation of extrinsic parameters – like generalized quantitative tear film deficiency or environmental stress and treatment modalities addressing these effects – can also be conducted using withdrawn organs and cell or organ cultures. An ex vivo model of dry eye was demonstrated for the first time by Choy et al. [4, 7], using freshly enucleated porcine eyes. Within this model, the variation in mimicked lacrimation and blinking intervals allows for the simulation of dry eye conditions of different levels of severity [28]. This model has already been applied to compare the effects of different artificial tears under simulated dry eye conditions [29]. Evaluation criteria accessible within this model are:

corneal damage (graded by fluorescein staining) and viability of cells in the central and peripheral region of the corneal epithelium (assessed by the trypan blue dye exclusion test after 4 h). Here, the time frame is limited by the increasing mortality rate of cells due to the reduction in their metabolic capabilities in the external environment.

To expand the usable time scale for experiments and to allow for a detailed analysis of corneal regeneration following corneal drying under different treatment conditions, it is feasible to apply corneal cultures as a substitute for the entire bulbi used by Choy et al. [4, 7, 28]. To reach this goal, we intend to integrate the established Ex Vivo Eye Irritation Test (EVEIT) into a model for DES, and in this report we present a feasible method for doing so. Fundamental experiments using time-resolved high-resolution optical coherence tomography (OCT) to investigate the initial behavior of the model under dry eye conditions are presented. Thereby, a detailed insight into the dynamic response of the cornea to different simulated lacrimation intervals is given. To demonstrate the capability of the combination of the introduced dry eye model and OCT examination, we additionally analyzed the effect of artificial tears applied under simulated dry eye conditions.

Materials and Methods

Ex Vivo Eye Irritation Test

The EVEIT allows for the prediction and grading of eye irritation and corrosion in chemical toxicology without the need for animal experiments [30]. This model is based on rabbit corneas slaughtered for food production. It has been proven to react very similarly to human eye tissue concerning behavior during chemical irritation and burn in single and repeated exposures. In a long-term approach, the self-healing system using organ culture methods (derived from human corneal culture) allows for an experimental time frame of up to 21 days. This enables the observation of biochemical and morphological changes after specific chemical exposures, including the evaluation of recovery after chemical or mechanical trauma. The healing process observed after mechanically induced epithelial damage within the EVEIT system is demonstrated in figure 1, using fluorescein staining for follow-up examination.

Engineered corneal tissue constructs tend to have a lack of epithelial integrity, permeability, and mechanical properties of the cornea [31]. The EVEIT system a priori contains the metabolic, functional and anatomical features of the living organ, and therefore there is no need to provide evidence of its similarity to natural cornea. The possibility of evaluating healing after corneal damage in vitro is a unique feature of the EVEIT [30] that will greatly enhance the prediction of pharmacological effectiveness using the intended DES model.

An alternative short-term approach of the EVEIT is performed on whole globes to investigate acute damage and penetration during chemical eye burn limited to a maximum observation period of approximately 6 h. Currently, the EVEIT is being further developed and standardized to meet the requirements for formal regulatory acceptance as a predictor of eye irritation.

Optical Coherence Tomography

In previous studies, it has been demonstrated that OCT is a valuable tool for evaluating morphological changes induced by the treatment conditions being tested and analyzing the process of recovery after chemical trauma within the EVEIT system [32, 33]. Compared to conventional his-

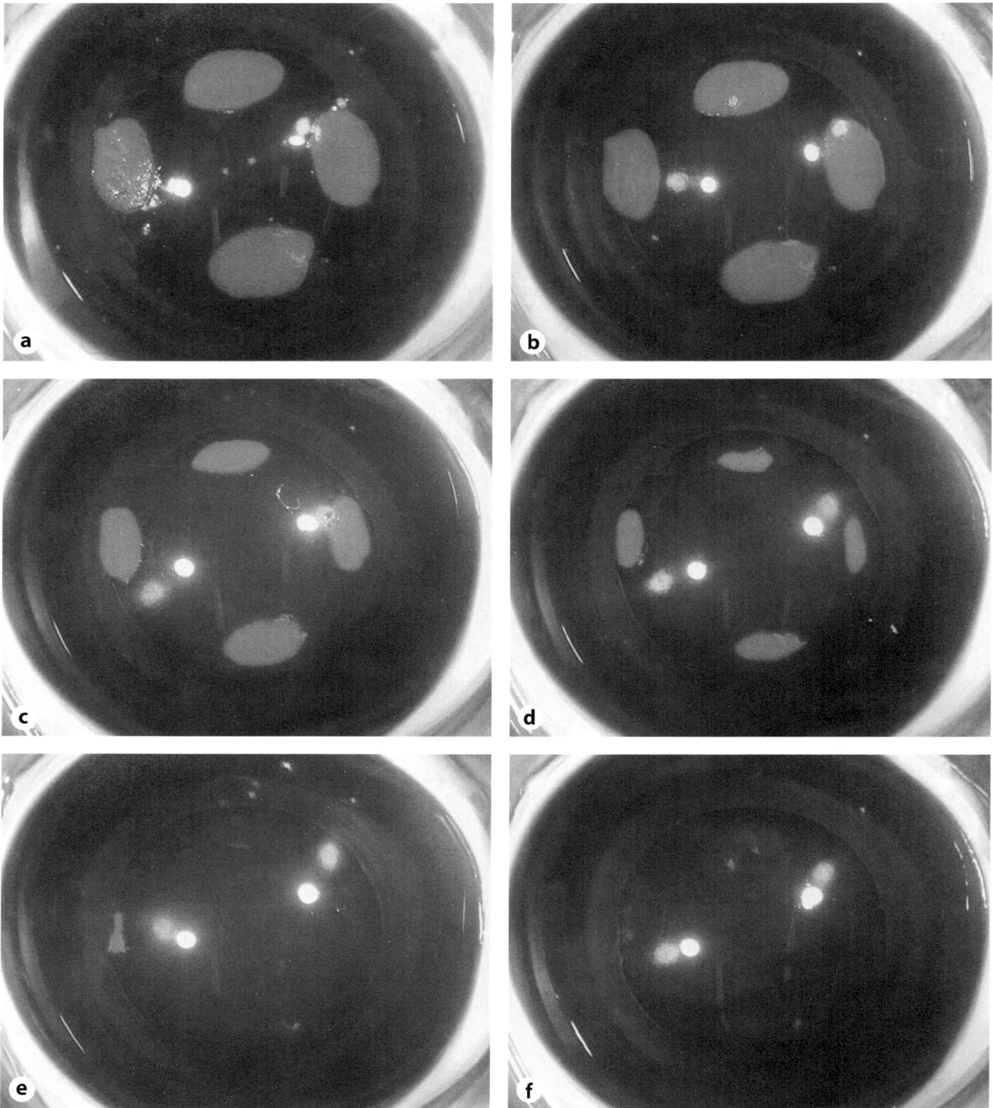

Fig. 1. Documentation of epithelial recovery, observed within the EVEIT system using fluorescein staining. Corneal culture imaged directly after epithelial abrasion in 4 areas, measuring approximately 4 mm² each (**a**). Images obtained 12 h (**b**), 24 h (**c**), 36 h (**d**), 48 h (**e**), and 60 h (**f**) after abrasion to document the healing process.

tological examination, this method enhances process monitoring from static invasive endpoint analysis to real-time dynamic observation. It therefore enables in situ monitoring of the area and the depth of damage, as well as recovery progress over time.

The basic principles of OCT have been extensively discussed elsewhere [34]. Briefly, OCT is the optical analog to medical sonography. For cross-sectional image reconstruction in OCT, near

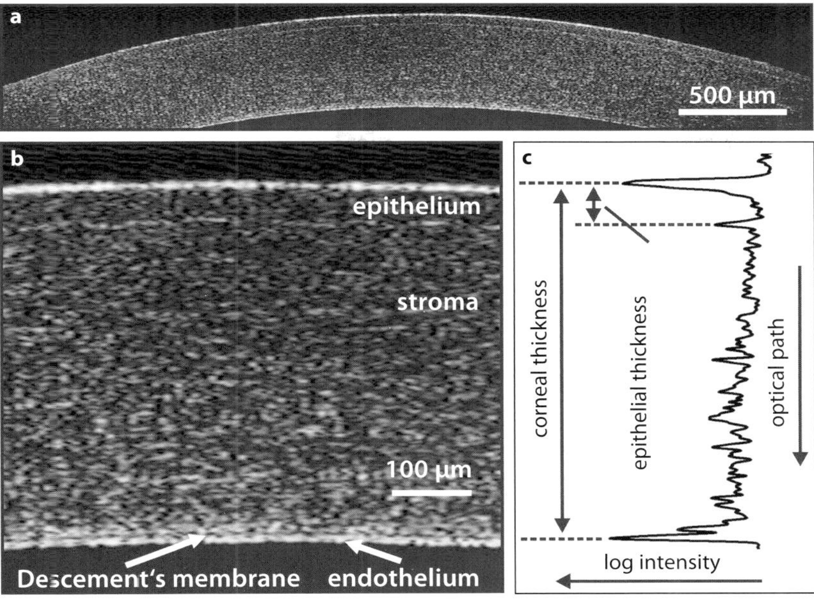

Fig. 2. High-resolution OCT image of an untreated rabbit cornea ex vivo. **a** Overview over the scanned region. 4,500 × 600 µm. **b** Magnification of the corneal apex. 600 × 600 µm. **c** Logarithmic intensity profile corresponding to **b** given by the average of 10 adjacent A-scans, demonstrating the entrance signals used to derive layer thicknesses.

infrared light (backscattered from structures within the sample) is analyzed by low-coherence interferometry. Hence, a light wave is split into a reference beam with variable path length and a probe beam, which is focused onto the sample. An interference signal is only generated if the path difference of both arms is smaller than the coherence length of the light source. Therefore, the axial resolution in OCT is determined by the coherence length, and consequently by the spectral bandwidth of the employed light source. In analogy to microscopy, the lateral resolution in OCT is determined by the cross-section of the laser beam at the sample site.

The high-resolution OCT system used in this study employs a Ti:sapphire laser oscillator (GigaJet 20, GigaOptics GmbH, Konstanz, Germany) centered at 800 nm as a low-coherence light source. Dispersion management within the laser cavity was deployed to optimize the coherence length of emitted light to 3.6 µm in air. The light source emission was coupled into the fiber-based interferometer of a commercial OCT system (Sirius 713, 4optics GmbH, Lübeck, Germany). The latter was modified to support the superior axial resolution specified by the coherence length of the Ti:sapphire laser. Axial and lateral resolutions within tissue were 2.6 and 10 µm, respectively. The A-scan rate of the OCT system was 50 Hz and the number of data points for each A-scan with an imaging depth of 600 µm was 512. A characteristic tomogram of an untreated rabbit cornea monitored by this OCT system is given in figure 2, demonstrating an overview of the scanned region (fig. 2a) and a magnification of the corneal apex (fig. 2b). Here, the epithelial and endothelial layers, the stroma, as well as Descement's membrane are distinguishable. Ten adjacent A-scans around the center of the image were averaged and plotted in figure 2c, representing the OCT signal amplitude on a logarithmic scale. Layer thicknesses of the cornea can be derived from the distances of the corresponding entrance signals. Here, the repeatability (defined as the standard deviation of

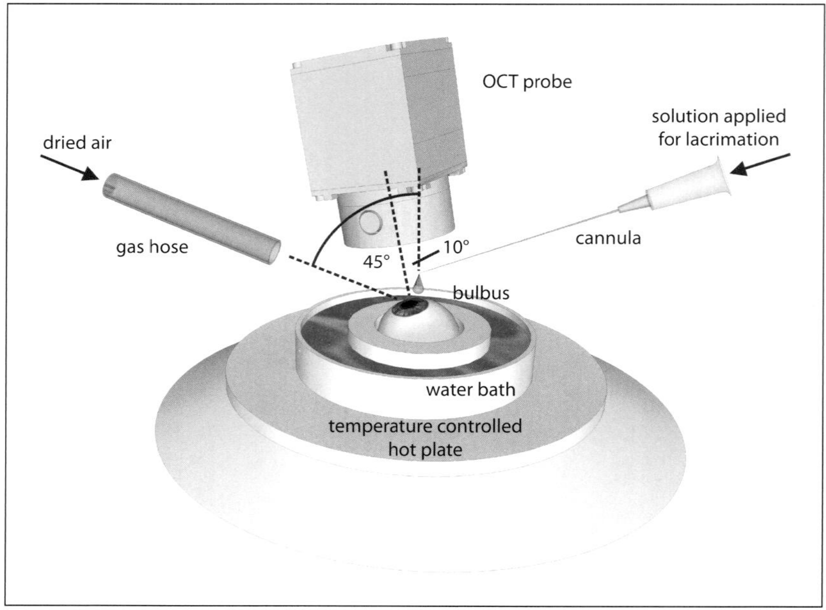

Fig. 3. Experimental setup used to investigate the desiccation of the cornea under simulated dry eye conditions.

the differences obtained in 5 independent and randomized measurements of epithelial thicknesses) was 1.76 μm, and therefore clearly below the axial resolution of the system.

Experimental Procedure

Within the research project described here, the short-term EVEIT was applied to define appropriate dry eye conditions to model different grades of dry eye. Additionally, the initial phase of corneal drying while simulating different lacrimation intervals and environmental conditions was studied. For this purpose, enucleated white rabbit eyes were used. Rabbit heads were obtained from an abattoir and kept cool until enucleation of the eyes. Only clear corneas without any epithelial defects were processed. All measurements were performed within 12 h after animal death. Excised globes were stored at 4°C within a moist chamber to ensure preservation of the corneal epithelium. Thirty minutes prior to measurements, all eyes were raised to a temperature of 32°C, corresponding to the corneal surface temperature observed in humans [35]. Corneal surface temperature was measured by an infrared thermometer, and was kept constant at 32 ± 2°C throughout the experiment by immersion of the posterior half of the bulbus into a temperature-controlled water bath (fig. 3). The bulbus was fixed within the water bath by a plastic ring with the cornea face up. Lacrimation was simulated by applying single drops of Ringer's solution (5.34 μl) at a defined interval onto the corneal surface. To this end, a cannula connected to a perfusion pump (IPC high-precision multichannel dispenser, Ismatec, Zürich, Switzerland) was placed above the cornea. By positioning the cannula relative to the cornea, an even distribution of the solution over the corneal epithelium was ensured. To simulate different environmental conditions, the humidity of the ambient air could be reduced by exchange with dried air at variable flow rate. For this purpose, a gas hose with internal diameter of 3.0 mm was used, as illustrated in figure 3. The distance from the nozzle to the corneal apex was 40 mm.

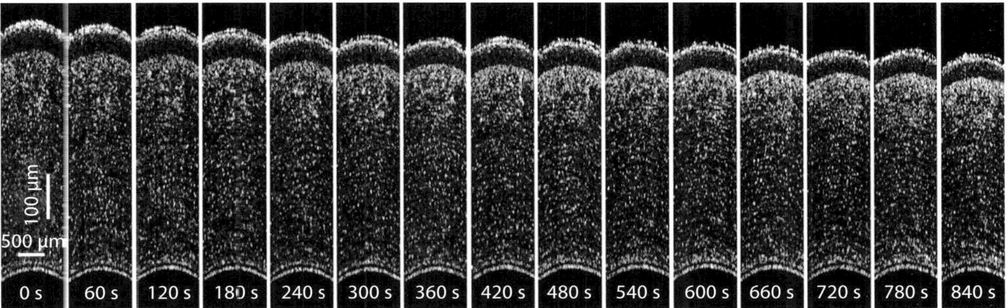

Fig. 4. OCT image sequence, obtained at a lacrimation interval of 60 s and a constant air flow of 2.0 l/min, demonstrating corneal desiccation under simulated dry eye conditions over a time period of 16 min. Each tomogram depicts a cross-sectional image of the cornea at the end of the respective lacrimation interval.

The development of corneal drying and the effect of simulated lacrimation on the corneal epithelium were monitored by OCT imaging with a frame rate of 15 tomograms per minute. The observation period of each run was 16 min, recording a total of 240 tomograms. All OCT measurements within this study were performed on the corneal apex (fig. 3). Tomograms applied for time-resolved measurements were composed of 167 A-scans with a lateral step size of 7 µm. Imaging was started directly after exposure of the cornea to ambient air, defining time point zero. Layer thicknesses of corneal epithelium and of the entire cornea were derived from the optical path lengths in between the corresponding entrance signals of epithelium and stroma on the one hand and epithelium and endothelium on the other hand, as demonstrated in figure 2c. A refractive index of 1.385 was assumed for the conversion of optical to geometrical path lengths [36].

Each experiment within this study was repeated twice, using enucleated eyes of different rabbits. Besides variations in the central corneal thickness of the untreated eyes in the range of 473 ± 30 µm and subsequent deviations in the observed corneal thicknesses during treatment, no significant variations in experimental outcome following identical treatment conditions were observed.

Results

Within our model, both the lacrimation interval and the humidity at the corneal surface can be varied to simulate different severities of dry eye. For the closely related model described by Choy et al. [4], which used enucleated porcine eyes, a lacrimation interval of 60 s is necessary to obtain a significant dry eye effect within a timeframe of 4 h. Here, air flow (not explicitly defined) was applied to increase the rate of evaporation on the corneal surface. To determine the effect of different magnitudes of the air flow, the initial phase of corneal desiccation was monitored by OCT at different flow rates using the short-term EVEIT.

Figure 4 shows a time-series data set obtained at a lacrimation interval of 60 s and a constant air flow of 2.0 l/min. Each tomogram depicts a cross-sectional image of the cornea at the end of the respective lacrimation interval. Two effects of the applied dry

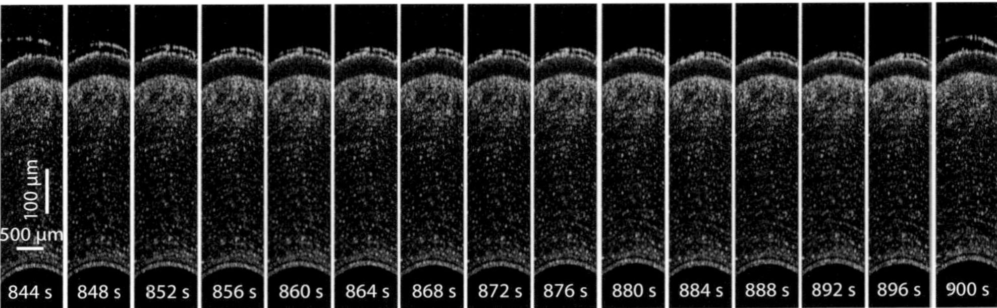

Fig. 5. OCT image sequence, obtained at a lacrimation interval of 60 s and a constant air flow of 2.0 l/min, demonstrating corneal reaction within a single lacrimation interval under simulated dry eye conditions.

eye conditions on the corneal structure can be seen in this time series: first, the corneal thickness decreases continuously with time; second, the OCT signal amplitude of the anterior stroma increases with time. Figure 5 illustrates the OCT images obtained during a single lacrimation interval within the same run depicted in figure 4. The first and the last tomograms within this series were recorded during the simulated lacrimation process, which becomes apparent from the liquid layer depicted on the surface of the epithelium. After application of Ringer's solution onto the corneal epithelium, the thickness of the liquid film decreased over time. However, at the end of the lacrimation interval, the liquid film still had a detectable thickness >3 µm. This finding holds true for all lacrimation intervals observed within this run, as is confirmed by the tomograms depicted in figure 4. Another important finding from the analysis of the lacrimation interval in figure 5 is the variation in epithelial thickness. In between 2 wetting procedures, simulating lacrimation at 60-second intervals, a continuous decrease in the layer thickness of the corneal epithelium was observed, whereas a rapid increase was found during the adjacent moistening procedure. A quantitative analysis of these findings is given in figure 6 for 3 runs recorded at different rates of dried air flow over the bulbus. Corneal and epithelial thicknesses were evaluated from the 240 tomograms obtained throughout each experiment and plotted against time. Vertical lines within the graphs define the current moments of corneal wetting as derived from OCT imaging. Here, minor deviations from the interval timer of the perfusion pump can be observed.

In figure 6a, measurements obtained without supplying dried air are analyzed. Measurements depicted in figure 6b and c were conducted at flow rates of 2.0 and 4.0 l/min, respectively. OCT data demonstrated in figures 4 and 5 are included in the diagram presented in figure 6b. In all these experiments, we observed a significant decrease in corneal thickness, which was determined to be 8.0, 16.3 and 44.7% of the initial thickness measured without air flow and flow rates of 2.0 and 4.0 l/min, respectively. Besides the continuous decrease in corneal thickness over time, an oscillation of corneal and epithelial thickness was observed on the timescale of

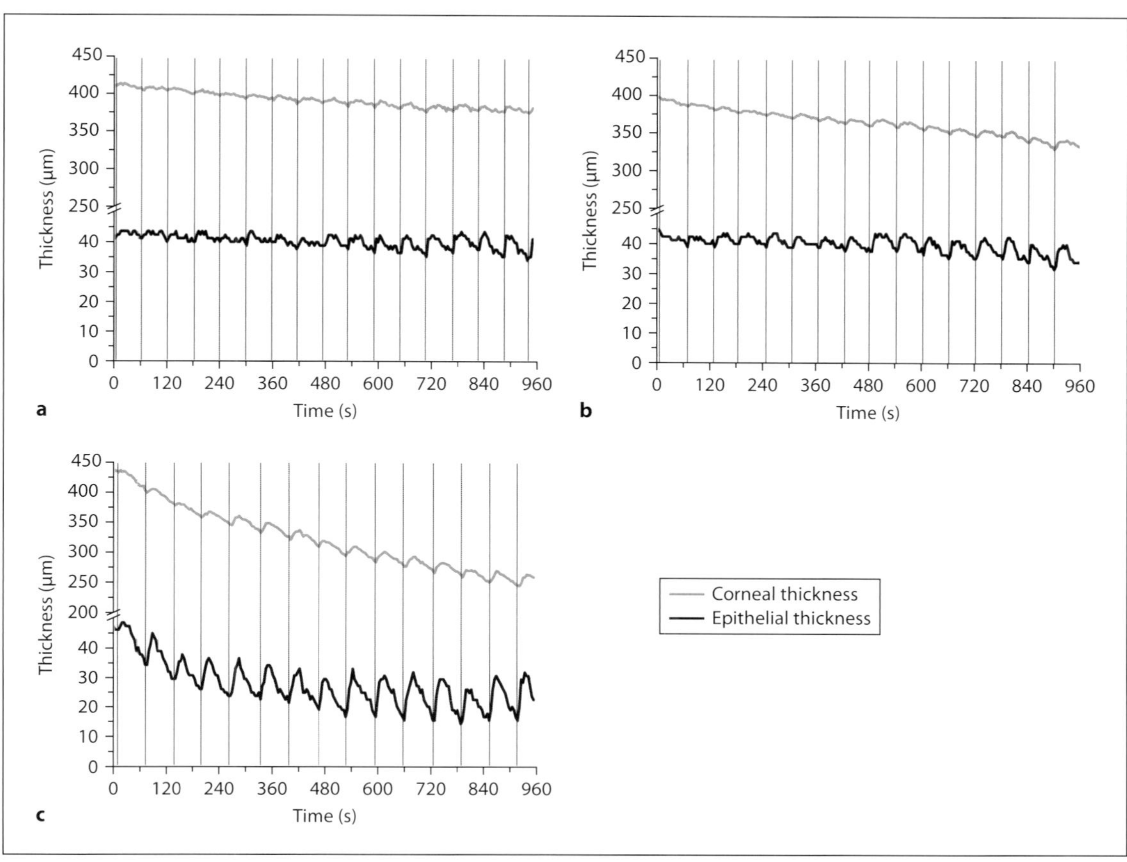

Fig. 6. Temporal development of corneal and epithelial thicknesses under simulated dry eye conditions derived from OCT time series. Vertical lines within the graphs indicate moments of simulated lacrimation. Values taken without supplying dried air (**a**), and at flow rates of 2.0 (**b**) and 4.0 l/min (**c**).

the lacrimation interval of approximately 60 s. Without air flow and with an air flow of only 2.0 l/min, the oscillation builds up during the observation period. Here, its amplitude exceeded the observational accuracy of the layer thicknesses only after 480 and 120 s, respectively.

The effect of artificial tears applied to the model under such simulated dry eye conditions is analyzed in figure 7. For corneal wetting, Hylocare® (Ursapharm GmbH, Saarbrücken, Germany) was used, which replaced Ringer's solution in the experiment depicted in figure 6b. By applying this highly viscous tear replacement solution at a lacrimation interval of 60 s in combination with an air flow of 2.0 l/min, a 6.9% decrease in corneal thickness was observed within 16 min. No variations in epithelial thickness exceeding the observational accuracy were observed within this time span.

To observe the effect of the lacrimation interval on the desiccation of the cornea, it was reduced to 20 s. This value has proven to be suitable to simulate non-desiccating

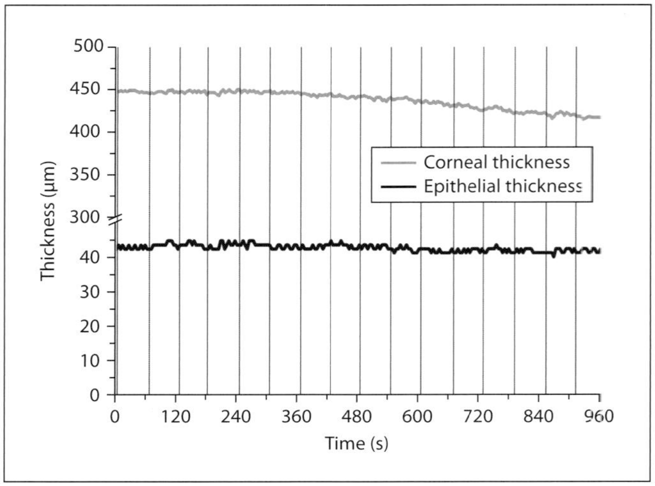

Fig. 7. Temporal development of corneal and epithelial thicknesses under simulated dry eye conditions (60-second lacrimation interval, 2.0 l/min flow rate of dried air) using artificial tears containing sodium hyaluronate. Vertical lines within the graphs indicate moments of simulated lacrimation.

conditions in the dry eye model of Choy et al. [4]. The air flow was adjusted to 2.0 l/min. Results obtained under these conditions within our system are presented in figure 8. Here, no variations in epithelial thickness exceeding the observational accuracy can be observed. Furthermore, the reduction of corneal thickness observed within 16 min is limited to 2.4% of the initial thickness. This is significantly less than the value of 16.3%, obtained for a lacrimation interval of 60 s under otherwise identical experimental conditions (fig. 6b).

Discussion

In this study, different evaporative conditions and intervals of simulated lacrimation have been studied in order to experimentally induce and treat dry eye symptoms using an in vitro model. High-resolution OCT provides objective information about the initial process of corneal desiccation, with different manifestations in the epithelium and stroma; thus, demonstrating that OCT is a valuable tool to adjust suitable conditions to model different severities of DES.

Time-resolved OCT imaging of corneal desiccation under dry eye conditions show an obvious increase in OCT signal amplitude in the anterior stroma over time, as given in figure 4. The OCT signal amplitude is determined by the scattering cross-section of the tissue under examination, and is therefore defined by its microstructure. Healthy corneal stroma transmits 99% of the incident light without scattering [37]. It is generally accepted that the fibril diameter, the interfibrillar distance and the lattice-like organization of the collagen fibrils play a crucial role in stromal transparency [38]. The observed increase in OCT signal amplitude can therefore be ascribed to structural changes in the anterior stroma, induced by a water flux to the corneal surface and subsequent stromal drying. This conclusion is supported by the observed decrease in corneal thickness over time. Figure 4 shows that the layer thickness of the tear film on the corneal surface clearly exceeded 3 μm during the entire experiment. As a result, under the applied conditions, corneal desiccation cannot be due to dry spots and evaporation directly on the corneal surface, but has to be accounted for by osmolar forces [39]. Evaporative removal of water from the tear film leads to an increase in osmolarity, and this in turn results in a detectable withdrawal of water from the stroma.

The main source of water in rabbit corneas is the free water within the tissue, which amounts to 76.3% of the corneal weight [40]. Removal of water from the anterior stroma results in increasing concentrations of salts within the cornea, leading to osmolarities of up to 600 mosm/kg measured in DES eyes. Thus, the water flux from the stroma to the corneal surface will decrease with decreasing difference in osmolarity. If the flux becomes to low to compensate for water loss in the epithelium, the epithelial thickness begins to oscillate at the lacrimation frequency, as demonstrated in figures 5 and 6, driven by the osmotic forces of the evaporating tear film. The observed rapid increase and slower decrease in thickness also supports this hypothesis, as a reduction in osmolarity is almost instantaneous when the tear substitute is applied, while evaporative increase in osmolarity is slow. In our model, such osmolar stress delivered to the epithelium was observed only after increased scattering in the anterior stroma was visualized in OCT imaging. Therefore, it can be concluded that water flux from the stroma to the epithelium can initially compensate osmolar desiccation of the epithelium.

The induced continuous change of swelling and shrinking is a membrane-destroying mechanism, resulting in surface damage of biological barriers, which is a typical clinical sign of dry eye, usually observed by fluorescein staining.

Reduced corneal thickness, as observed in our model system, has been assessed as a target variable in dry eye therapy by Karadayi et al. [41]. They documented corneal thicknesses before and after therapy of dry eye patients with tear substitutes. This study confirmed a mean increase in corneal thickness of 29 μm for patients with DES after 2 weeks of therapy. For normal individuals, lacking any symptoms of DES, the mean increase was only 3 μm. Clinical studies on trachomatous dry eyes and on DES have confirmed that corneal thinning is a valuable clinical sign of DES [42, 43]. This fact can easily be incorporated into our dry eye model using OCT for follow-up observation, e.g. in therapeutic studies.

In the normal eye, one third of the tear flow evaporates. However, in dry eye, up to three quarters of the tear film evaporates depending on the distinct pathological entity [44, 45]. Because evaporation accounts for a significant proportion of the tear loss in patients with dry eye, it also plays a crucial role in modeling of DES. Assuming constant temperatures of tear film and surrounding air, the evaporation rate is inversely proportional to relative humidity. This was used to study the influence of tear evaporation on the initial process of corneal desiccation by applying dried air at different flow rates at the corneal surface (fig. 6). Here, measurements without air flow (fig. 6a) and with an air flow of 2.0 l/min (fig 6b) can be described as combined tear deficient and evaporative dry eye conditions. These are characterized by a preceding desiccation of the anterior stroma and subsequent alternating shrinkage and swelling of the epithelial layer, driven by osmotic forces of the evaporating tear film, as discussed earlier. The higher evaporation rate, which takes place when dried air is applied, only results in quantitative differences concerning the rates of stroma desiccation and corneal shrinkage and is subsequent to the point in time when significant oscillation of the epithelial thickness is observed.

At even higher evaporation rates, the tear film break-up time is less than 60 s, and therefore below the lacrimation interval applied. At an air flow of 4 l/min, tear film break-up time can be estimated from OCT data to be 32 s (not shown here). In this case, epithelial damage is not only driven by osmolar forces, but also by evaporative desiccation of the epithelial cells. This is apparent in the instantaneous and irreversible shrinkage of the epithelial layer observed under these conditions (fig. 6c). Such severe evaporative conditions are not adequate to induce dry eye conditions, and consequently will be avoided in further studies. This is justified by the fact that blinking is especially controlled by ocular surface conditions, resulting in an increased blink rate below the tear film break-up time for dry eye patients with normal corneal sensitivity [46, 47].

Within the first experimental application of our method in pharmacological screening, repeated use of hyaluronate-containing eye drops under simulated severe dry eye conditions was investigated. Application of such a tear replacement solution clearly showed a significant reduction in stained epithelial cells in the trypan blue exclusion test using the porcine dry eye model of Choy et al. [29]. This finding could be reproduced successfully by our model; thus, providing initial confirmation of the applicability of the presented dry eye model in pharmacological tests. It can be concluded from the obtained OCT data that application of this artificial tear replacement prevents the epithelium from being exposed to osmotic stress (fig. 7), while the opposite is observed for application of Ringer's solution as a tear replacement under the same conditions (fig. 6b). Two reasons can be attributed to this finding. First, the water-binding capacity of sodium hyaluronate may increase the water content of the epithelium; second, the high viscosity of the fluid which increases the contact time on the corneal surface.

For use as a negative control, simulation of normal tear film conditions is also important. This is achieved using higher lacrimation rates, as demonstrated in figure 8. Here, stromal desiccation and thereby corneal shrinkage are clearly reduced. In particular, no change in epithelial thickness is observed. Thus, it can be concluded that evaporation within the timeframe of 20 s does not lead to excessive osmolarities of the tear film. Accordingly, no damage to the corneal epithelium induced by osmolar stress is expected under these conditions.

Fig. 8. Temporal development of corneal and epithelial thicknesses under simulated normal conditions (20-second lacrimation interval, 2.0 l/min flow rate of dried air) derived from OCT time series. Vertical lines within the graphs indicate moments of simulated lacrimation.

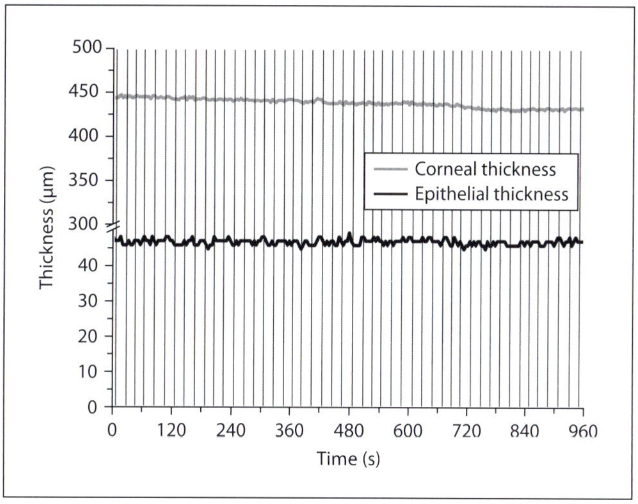

The results obtained in this preliminary study form a solid basis to further develop the dry eye model introduced here. An important next step will be the transition from the short-term to the long-term approach using the corneal culture system established within the EVEIT. As the time in which the cornea is exposed to dry eye conditions is a key factor for the induced corneal damage, it will be necessary to adapt the environmental conditions for taking this step. For example, it will be necessary to investigate whether a further reduction in the lacrimation interval below 20 s is required to simulate normal conditions over a period of several days. Here, OCT monitoring will be a valuable tool to adjust these conditions, as it supplies not only information about the corneal desiccation, but also gives a detailed insight into the osmotic processes which introduce this stromal and epithelial damage.

Conclusion

There is no doubt that a meaningful in vitro dry eye model will achieve widespread use in order to address scientific problems and develop new treatment strategies and diagnostic approaches for DES. First important steps towards this goal have already been demonstrated within the research project described here, including an applicable corneal culture system, dynamic OCT monitoring of corneal response to the applied dry eye conditions, and adjustable experimental conditions to model different severities of DES. Combining the introduced short-term approach of the dry eye model with the presented corneal culture system will be the next step towards a new and innovative dry eye model. This will allow, for the first time, investigation of the healing processes under simulated dry eye conditions in vitro.

Acknowledgment

We gratefully acknowledge scientific contributions by Stefan Kray and Jaroslav Lazar. This work was partially funded by the Federal Ministry of Education and Research (BMBF), grants 0315491A and 0315491B and by a Pathfinder project within the Exploratory Research Space (ERS) @ RWTH Aachen, grant OPPa71.

References

1 Schrage N, Wuestemeyer H, Langefeld S: Do different osmolar solutions change the epithelial surface of the healthy rabbit cornea? Graefes Arch Clin Exp Ophthalmol 2004;242:668–673.
2 Schrader S, Mircheff AK, Geerling G: Animal models of dry eye. Dev Ophthalmol 2008;41:298–312.
3 Virtanen T, Konttinen YT, Honkanen N, Härkönen M, Tervo T: Tear fluid plasmin activity of dry eye patients with Sjögren's syndrome. Acta Ophthalmol Scand 1997;75:137–141.
4 Choy EP, Cho P, Benzie IF, Choy CK, To TS: A novel porcine dry eye model system (pDEM) with simulated lacrimation/blinking system: preliminary findings on system variability and effect of corneal drying. Curr Eye Res 2004;28:319–325.
5 Dursun D, Wang M, Monroy D, Li DQ, Lokeshwar BL, Stern ME, Pflugfelder SC: A mouse model of keratoconjunctivitis sicca. Invest Ophthalmol Vis Sci 2002;43:632–638.
6 Terry MA: Dry eye in the elderly. Drugs Aging 2001; 18:101–107.
7 Choy EP, To TS, Cho P, Benzie IF, Choy CK: Viability of porcine corneal epithelium ex vivo and effect of exposure to air: a pilot study for a dry eye model. Cornea 2004;23:715–719.
8 Brewitt H, Sistani F: Dry eye disease: the scale of the problem. Surv Ophthalmol 2001;45(suppl 2):S199–S202.
9 Schein OD, Muñoz B, Tielsch JM, Bandeen-Roche K, West S: Prevalence of dry eye among the elderly. Am J Ophthalmol 1997;124:723–728.
10 McCarty CA, Bansal AK, Livingston PM, Stanislavsky YL, Taylor HR: The epidemiology of dry eye in Melbourne, Australia. Ophthalmology 1998;105: 1114–1119.
11 Lin PY, Tsai SY, Cheng CY, Liu JH, Chou P, Hsu WM: Prevalence of dry eye among an elderly Chinese population in Taiwan: the Shihpai Eye Study. Ophthalmology 2003;110:1096–1101.
12 Wolkoff P, Kjaergaard SK: The dichotomy of relative humidity on indoor air quality. Environ Int 2007;33: 850–857.
13 Segal B, Bowman SJ, Fox PC, Vivino FB, Murukutla N, Brodscholl J, Ogale S, McLean L: Primary Sjögren's syndrome: health experiences and predictors of health quality among patients in the United States. Health Qual Life Outcomes 2009;7:46.
14 Kunert KS, Tisdale AS, Stern ME, Smith JA, Gipson IK: Analysis of topical cyclosporine treatment of patients with dry eye syndrome: effect on conjunctival lymphocytes. Arch Ophthalmol 2000;118:1489–1496.
15 Stern ME, Gao J, Schwalb TA, Ngo M, Tieu DD, Chan CC, Reis BL, Whitcup SM, Thompson D, Smith JA: Conjunctival T-cell subpopulations in Sjögren's and non-Sjögren's patients with dry eye. Invest Ophthalmol Vis Sci 2002;43:2609–2614.
16 Liu Z, Pflugfelder SC: Corneal surface regularity and the effect of artificial tears in aqueous tear deficiency. Ophthalmology 1999;106:939–943.
17 Behrens A, Doyle JJ, Stern L, Chuck RS, McDonnell PJ, Azar DT, Dua HS, Hom M, Karpecki PM, Laibson PR, Lemp MA, Meisler DM, Del Castillo JM, O'Brien TP, Pflugfelder SC, Rolando M, Schein OD, Seitz B, Tseng SC, van Setten G, Wilson SE, Yiu SC: Dysfunctional tear syndrome: a Delphi approach to treatment recommendations. Cornea 2006;25:900–907.
18 Foulks GN: The correlation between the tear film lipid layer and dry eye disease. Surv Ophthalmol 2007;52:369–374.
19 Barabino S, Dana MR: Animal models of dry eye: a critical assessment of opportunities and limitations. Invest Ophthalmol Vis Sci 2004;45:1641–1646.
20 Zhu L, Shen J, Zhang C, Park CY, Kohanim S, Yew M, Parker JS, Chuck RS: Inflammatory cytokine expression on the ocular surface in the Botulium toxin B induced murine dry eye model. Mol Vis 2009;15:250–258.
21 Helper LC, Magrane WG, Koehm J, Johnson R: Surgical induction of keratoconjunctivitis sicca in the dog. J Am Vet Med Assoc 1974;165:172–174.

22 Hakim SG, Schroder C, Geerling G, Lauer I, Wedel T, Kosmehl H, Driemel O, Jacobsen HC, Trenkle T, Hermes D, Sieg P: Early and late immunohistochemical and ultrastructural changes associated with functional impairment of the lachrymal gland following external beam radiation. Int J Exp Pathol 2006;87:65–71.
23 Gilbard JP, Rossi SR, Gray KL, Hanninen LA, Kenyon KR: Tear film osmolarity and ocular surface disease in two rabbit models for keratoconjunctivitis sicca. Invest Ophthalmol Vis Sci 1988;29:374–378.
24 Fujihara T, Nagano T, Nakamura M, Shirasawa E: Lactoferrin suppresses loss of corneal epithelial integrity in a rabbit short-term dry eye model. J Ocul Pharmacol Ther 1998;14:99–107.
25 Fabiani C, Barabino S, Rashid S, Dana MR: Corneal epithelial proliferation and thickness in a mouse model of dry eye. Exp Eye Res 2009;89:166–171.
26 Nakamura S, Shibuya M, Nakashima H, Hisamura R, Masuda N, Imagawa T, Uehara M, Tsubota K: Involvement of oxidative stress on corneal epithelial alterations in a blink-suppressed dry eye. Invest Ophthalmol Vis Sci 2007;48:1552–1558.
27 Drummond PD: Lacrimation and cutaneous vasodilatation in the face induced by painful stimulation of the nasal ala and upper lip. J Auton Nerv Syst 1995;51:109–116.
28 Choy EP, Cho P, Benzie IF, Choy CK: Dry eye and blink rate simulation with a pig eye model. Optom Vis Sci 2008;85:129–134.
29 Choy EP, Cho P, Benzie IF, Choy CK: Investigation of corneal effect of different types of artificial tears in a simulated dry eye condition using a novel porcine dry eye model (pDEM). Cornea 2006;25:1200–1204.
30 Frentz M, Goss M, Reim M, Schrage NF: Repeated exposure to benzalkonium chloride in the Ex Vivo Eye Irritation Test (EVEIT): observation of isolated corneal damage and healing. Altern Lab Anim 2008;36:25–32.
31 Berry M, Radburn-Smith M: Ocular toxicology in vitro – cell based assays. ALTEX 2006;23(suppl):313–317.
32 Spöler F, Först M, Kurz H, Frentz M, Schrage NF: Dynamic analysis of chemical eye burns using high-resolution optical coherence tomography. J Biomed Opt 2007;12:041203.
33 Spöler F, Frentz M, Först M, Kurz H, Schrage NF: Analysis of hydrofluoric acid penetration and decontamination of the eye by means of time-resolved optical coherence tomography. Burns 2008;34:549–555.
34 Fercher AF, Drexler W, Hitzenberger CK, Lasser T: Optical coherence tomography – principles and applications. Rep Prog Phys 2003;66:239–303.
35 Schrage NF, Flick S, von Fischern T, Reim M, Wenzel M: Temperature changes of the cornea by applying an eye bandage. Ophthalmologe 1997;94:492–495.
36 Drexler W, Hitzenberger CK, Baumgartner A, Findl O, Sattmann H, Fercher AF: Investigation of dispersion effects in ocular media by multiple wavelength partial coherence interferometry. Exp Eye Res 1998;66:25–33.
37 Meek KM, Leonard DW: Ultrastructure of the corneal stroma: a comparative study. Biophys J 1993;64:273–280.
38 Meek KM, Boote C: The organization of collagen in the corneal stroma. Exp Eye Res 2004;78:503–512.
39 Mishima S, Maurice DM: The effect of normal evaporation on the eye. Exp Eye Res 1961;1:46–52.
40 von Fischern T, Lorenz U, Burchard WG, Reim M, Schrage NF: Changes in mineral composition of rabbit corneas after alkali burn. Graefes Arch Clin Exp Ophthalmol 1998;236:553–558.
41 Karadayi K, Ciftci F, Akin T, Bilge AH: Increase in central corneal thickness in dry and normal eyes with application of artificial tears: a new diagnostic and follow-up criterion for dry eye. Ophthalmic Physiol Opt 2005;25:485–491.
42 Guzey M, Satici A, Karadede S: Corneal thickness in trachomatous dry eye. Eur J Ophthalmol 2002;12:18–23.
43 Liu Z, Pflugfelder SC: Corneal thickness is reduced in dry eye. Cornea 1999;18:403–407.
44 Mathers WD, Daley TE: Tear flow and evaporation in patients with and without dry eye. Ophthalmology 1996;103:664–669.
45 Goto E, Matsumoto Y, Kamoi M, Endo K, Ishida R, Dogru M, Kaido M, Kojima T, Tsubota K: Tear evaporation rates in Sjögren syndrome and non-Sjögren dry eye patients. Am J Ophthalmol 2007;144:81–85.
46 Nakamori K, Odawara M, Nakajima T, Mizutani T, Tsubota K: Blinking is controlled primarily by ocular surface conditions. Am J Ophthalmol 1997;124:24–30.
47 Nally L, Ousler GW, Emory TB, Abelson MB: A correlation between blink rate and corneal sensitivity in a dry eye population. Invest Ophthalmol Vis Sci 2003;44:E-abstract 2488.

Dr. rer. nat. Felix Spöler
Institute of Semiconductor Electronics, RWTH Aachen University
Sommerfeldstrasse 24
DE–52074 Aachen (Germany)
Tel. +49 241 80 27896, Fax +49 241 80 22246, E-Mail spoeler@iht.rwth-aachen.de

Brewitt H (ed): Research Projects in Dry Eye Syndrome.
Dev Ophthalmol. Basel, Karger, 2010, vol 45, pp 108–122

The Lid Margin Is an Underestimated Structure for Preservation of Ocular Surface Health and Development of Dry Eye Disease

Erich Knop[a] · Donald R. Korb[b] · Caroline A. Blackie[b] · Nadja Knop[c]

[a]Research Laboratory, Department of Ophthalmology CVK, Charité – Universitätsmedizin Berlin, Berlin, Germany; [b]Korb Associates, Boston, Mass., USA; [c]Department of Cell Biology in Anatomy, Hannover Medical School, Hannover, Germany

Abstract

Purpose: The structure of the lid margin is insufficiently understood and defined, although it is of obvious importance in ocular surface integrity. **Methods:** The structure and function of the different zones of the lid margin are explained with a focus on dry eye disease. **Results:** The posterior lid margin, which is of particular significance for the integrity of the ocular surface, includes the meibomian glands that open within the cornified epidermis. Their obstructive dysfunction is a main cause of dry eye disease. The orifice is followed by the mucocutaneous junction, which extends from the abrupt termination of the epidermis to the crest of the inner lid border. The physiological vital stainable line of Marx represents its surface, and can be used e.g. as a diagnostic tool for the location and functionality of the meibomian gland orifices and lacrimal puncta. The marginal conjunctiva starts at the crest of the inner lid border and forms a thickened epithelial cushion. This is the point closest to the globe, and represents the zone that wipes the bulbar surface and distributes the thin preocular tear film. It is hence termed the 'lid wiper' and pathological alterations that result in a vital staining are a sensitive early indicator of dry eye disease. **Conclusions:** The margin of the eyelid is an important but currently underestimated structure in the maintenance of the preocular tear film and of the utmost importance for the preservation of ocular surface integrity and in the development of dry eye disease.

Introduction

The Lid Margin Is an Important but Currently Underestimated Structure

The margin of the eye lid is an essential structure in the maintenance of preocular tear film and of the utmost importance to the functional anatomy of the ocular surface [1] for the preservation of its integrity. Lid margin dysfunction is also an important factor in the development of dry eye disease [2–7].

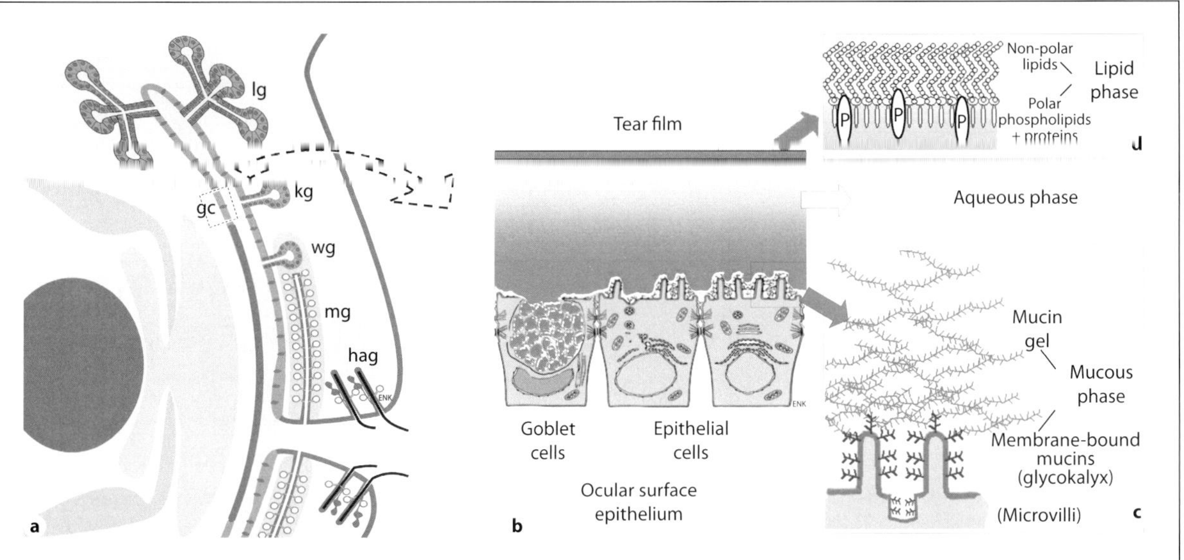

Fig. 1. Glands of the ocular surface and preocular tear film. **a** Several glands that are either located directly at the ocular surface or connected to it via their excretory duct contribute to the production of the tear film. The aqueous phase is produced by the main lacrimal gland (lg) that is located in the orbit and delivers its fluid via multiple excretory ducts into the conjunctival fornix, by the accessory lacrimal glands located in the orbital tissue (Krause glands, kg) and in the proximal part of the tarsus (Wolfring glands, wg). The mucin layer is produced by the goblet cells (gc) inside the conjunctival and by the conventional conjunctival epithelial cells; the lipid phase is produced by the large tarsal glands of Meibom (mg) inside the tarsal plates that deliver their oily secretion through a short excretory duct at the posterior lid margin onto the tear meniscus. At the anterior lid margin, there are also hair-associated glands (hag) of Zeis and Moll. **b** The tear film is principally thought to form 3 layers that mix to a certain degree. **c** The mucus phase consists of the membrane-bound glycocalyx of the ordinary epithelial cells of the ocular surface epithelia, located on their microvilli, and of the gel-forming mucins from the goblet cells. The gel-forming mucins increasingly mix and dilute within the overlying aqueous phase. This mucinous-aqueous phase constitutes the main part of the tear film and is provided with a superficial thin layer of lipids. **d** Within this, polar lipids and potentially proteins maintain the binding of the overlying non-polar lipids which can not directly mix with water. The exact conformation, composition and thickness of the tear film and its layers, particularly the lipid layer, is still under debate. Reproduced from E. Knop et al. [1] with permission from Springer.

The importance of the lid margin is apparently underestimated at present because research focused on ocular surface integrity and tears has usually been centered around the source of the tear fluid derived from the secretion of the ocular-surface-associated glands, i.e. the lacrimal gland, accessory lacrimal glands, goblet cells that are interspersed in the conjunctiva, and the meibomian glands inside the tarsal plates of the eyelids (fig. 1a). The latter contribute the superficial lipid layer to the tear film, but have received only limited attention clinically and scientifically. This has only recently begun to change with the recognition that alterations in the lipid phase [8] caused by meibomian gland dysfunction (in particular of the obstructive type [9]) are a main cause of dry eyes.

Another area of focus has been the equipment of the ocular surface epithelia with lubricative mucins that contribute to the adherence of aqueous tears [10] (fig. 1b, c) [11, 12]. This attention on mucins historically derives from early observations that seemed to show [13] that the corneal surface is non-wettable and could only be lubricated through coating with mucins [14]. Also the formation of dry spots, as an early sign of tear film deterioration and dry eye condition, was related to a local mucin deficiency [15].

Functions of the Lid Margin

The Lid Margin Preserves Ocular Surface Integrity

In contrast to these conventional considerations, the lid margin represents the 'other end' of the tears and appears to be equally important for ocular surface lubrication; it conceivably has several functions: (1) acting as a static dam, since the inner lid margin limits the tear lake (meniscus) and hence prevents the potential loss of tears from the ocular surface by spillage over the anterior lid border and guides the tear flow along the lid margin towards the lacrimal puncta [16, 17]; (2) distributing tears (posterior lid border) [18] in a way comparable with a windscreen wiper [19] because with every blink the movement of the lid margin guarantees the required thin expansion of the tear film in order to form a thin optically perfect tissue-air interface [4, 20–22]; (3) coating the thin tear film with oil of the tarsal meibomian glands (delivered anterior to the meniscus), and thus preventing evaporation of the aqueous phase [23–26]; (4) meibomian oil presumably prevents the skin lipids (found to induce tear film rupture [27]) entering the tear film.

Alterations in the Lid Margin Are Associated with Ocular Surface Disease

Clinically, it is well known that deterioration of the lid margin is often associated with ocular surface disease [28–34]. Surprisingly, however, the microanatomy of the different regions of the human lid margin has been poorly defined, which results in difficulties in describing normal morphology and its alterations in disease states. Clinically, the whole lid margin is usually addressed just as the 'margin' and subzones are not specifically differentiated (e.g. free *margin* versus anterior or posterior *border*).

If the mucocutaneous junction (MCJ) is considered, this is often thought to extend onto the tarsal side [35], and the nature and localization of the line of Marx have remained enigmatic for a long time. The zonal differentiation at the inner lid border is currently unclear with respect to the MCJ, the line of Marx and the lid wiper. Since this region is of the utmost importance for the continuous distribution and reformation of the preocular tear film with every blink, it conceivably has eminent implications for ocular surface health and integrity as well as for the development of dry eye disease. This also applies to the morphological changes that underlie the development of obstructive meibomian gland dysfunction, which appears to represent the single most frequent cause of dry eye disease [9].

The current knowledge and the remaining unresolved issues of lid margin anatomy and function that are relevant for understanding dry eye disease will be explained and discussed in this contribution.

Structures at the Lid Margin and Their Involvement in Dry Eye Disease

Anatomy and Pathology of the Meibomian Glands

The meibomian glands, also termed tarsal glands of Meibom (glandulae tarsales) because of their location inside the tarsal plates, are large sebaceous glands in the eyelids with no association to hairs. Pathological alterations in the meibomian glands, which are mainly summarized as 'meibomian gland dysfunction' (MGD) [36], are increasingly being recognized as a discrete disease entity [30, 37] and an important factor in evaporative dry eye disease [8, 9]. The meibomian glands are single glands that open at the posterior lid margin (fig. 2a) close to the termination of the cornified epidermis, but are usually still encircled by epidermis. The glands can be seen as white-to-yellowish structures underneath the conjunctiva throughout the length of the tarsal plates in the upper and lower lids when the lid is everted (fig. 2b) or visualized by transillumination. Numerous secretory acini are arranged around the long central duct and connected to it by small ductules (fig. 3c). Many of these separate glands are arranged in a sheet that almost completely fills the extension of the tarsal plates [38–41].

Meibomian Ductal System Shows Signs of Incipient Keratinization

The holocrine secretory acini of the meibomian glands have a longish-to-roundish shape and are completely filled with pale secretory cells, which are termed meibocytes [42] (fig. 3a). They produce and accumulate lipids inside the cell until they degenerate and release their entire cell contents which form the meibomian oil (meibum) [42]. The oil is released through the connecting ductule into the long central duct (fig. 2c), which are both lined by a 4-layer stratified squamous epithelium [41].

The terminal part of the central duct has a different structure and is formed by an ingrowth of the epidermis from the free lid margin; it must therefore be separately designated from the rest of the central duct as an excretory duct. The excretory duct is lined by epidermis that loses the cornification after about half a millimeter, by loss of the keratin lamellae and the granular layer, and transforms into the usual 4-layer stratified squamous epithelium of the ductal system. Around the terminal part of the gland (excretory duct, the terminal part of the central duct and terminal acini) close to the free lid margin, there are varying amounts of striated fibers of Riolan's muscle (fig. 2c, 3b, d) [41, 43, 44] which are split from the orbicularis muscle by the downgrowth of the cilia deep into the tarsal fold during embryological development [19].

Interestingly, recent investigations have shown that in fact the whole ductal epithelium of the normal human meibomian gland has preserved a certain degree of

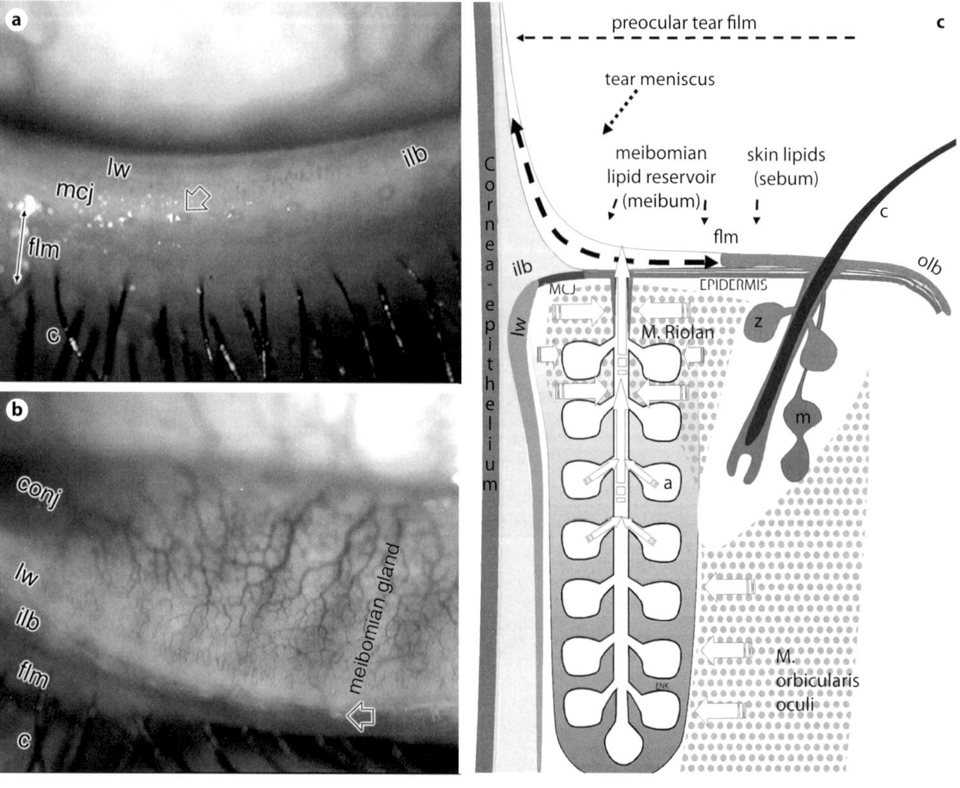

Fig. 2. Zones and structures of the human lid margin. The lid margin consists of different zones with differential structure as seen in photomicrographs that show a lid margin in a slightly (**a**) and in a strongly (**b**) everted position as well as in a schematic drawing (**c**). From distal to proximal, the cornified stratified squamous epithelium of the skin (epidermis) extends from the outer skin of the lid over the outer lid border (olb). It grows deep into the lid body to give rise to the ciliary hair follicles and their associated glands of Zeis (z) and Moll (ml). It covers the free lid margin (flm), grows deep again to provide the origin of the meibomian glands, and also typically encircles the orifices of the meibomian glands (open arrows). The MCJ is located proximal to the epidermal cuff around the orifices of the meibomian glands at the inner lid border (ilb) and is followed by the lid wiper (lw), which represents the initial thickening of the conjunctival mucosal epithelium and serves as a device to spread the tear fluid from the marginal tear meniscus into the thin preocular tear film during the up-phase of every blink. The aqueous tear fluid is covered by a thin outer layer of lipids that are produced by the meibomian glands inside the tarsal plate of the lid. Lipids are produced by the numerous roundish holocrine sebaceous acini (a) in the gland periphery, then transported (small white arrows) through the connecting ductules into the long central duct and delivered through a short excretory duct and orifice onto the posterior lid margin. The driving forces for the delivery of meibum are the constant secretory force together with the mechanical action (large white arrows) of the orbicularis muscle (orb) and the muscle of Riolan at the posterior lid margin that occur with every blink. Reproduced from E. Knop et al. [37a, 37b] with permission from Springer.

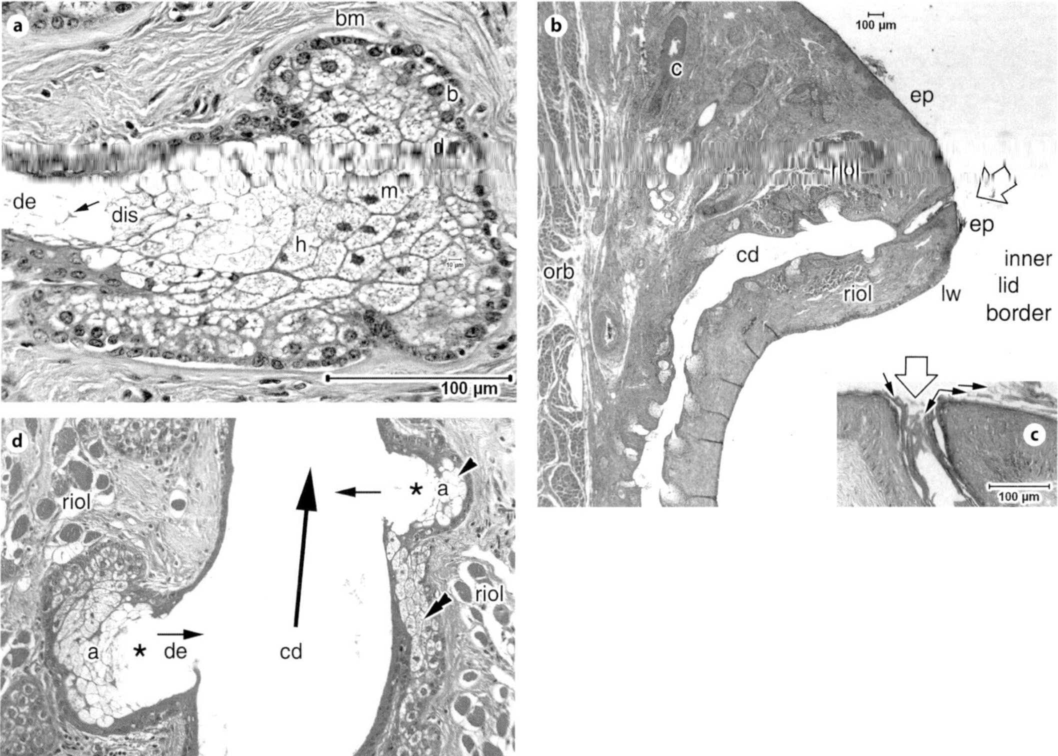

Fig. 3. Structure of the acini and ductal system of the meibomian gland. **a** Holocrine acinus of a normal meibomian gland filled with secretory cells (meibocytes) and surrounded by a basement membrane (bm). From the basal cells (b) at the periphery, differentiating (d), meibocytes start with the production and accumulation of lipids within droplets and move towards the acinus center leading to large mature (m) meibocytes. The very large hypermature (h) meibocytes, disintegrate (dis) and their entire cell contents form the oily secretory product (termed meibum) close to the connecting ductule (de). Remnants (arrow) of the meibocytes are still found inside the ductule. **b** An obstructed Meibomian gland shows signs of degeneration due to the increased internal pressure. The central duct (cd) is partly dilated and slightly undulated. **c** The orifice (open arrow) is obstructed by accumulations of cornified keratin lamellae (filled arrows). **d** Under higher magnification, the epithelium that lines the dilated central duct (cd) is seen to be compressed, the connecting ductules (de) are widened, the acini (a) are reduced in size and degenerated. Their secretory cells (meibocytes) are reduced in number to a few layers of bright cells in the periphery (arrowhead). Occasionally residual degenerated acini are embedded into the wall of the central duct (double arrowheads) HE.

incipient keratinization, as verified by the regular presence of keratohyalin granules in the luminal epithelial cell layer [45]. This can be explained by the similarity in structure and embryological development of the meibomian glands to the ciliary hair follicles [reviewed in 41], and it also explains why hyperkeratinization is a typical pathology that leads to MGD.

Hyperkeratinization Is a Major Cause of Obstructive MGD and Results in Degenerative Gland Dilatation and Atrophy
Obstructive MGD due to hyperkeratinization was first described in patients with only minimal or transient symptoms suggestive of ocular dryness who became clinically symptomatic due to a contact lens intolerance. Manual expression of their meibomian glands revealed clusters of desquamated hyperkeratotic epithelial cells embedded in a thickened meibum that had obstructed the orifices, and histology verified a dilatation of the central duct by such material [36]. After expression and removal of theses plugs, the tear film normalized and contact lens intolerance disappeared [46]. Later histological examinations of the meibomian glands from patients with symptomatic dry eye disease, which showed inspissation of orifices and expressible highly viscous secretion, verified obstruction of the excretory duct by increased keratinization. Inside the gland, this had resulted in dilatation of the ductal system as well as enlargement of acini with cystic degeneration, loss of secretory meibocytes (fig. 3b, d) and their replacement by a squamous metaplasia [47].

Obstructive MDG Results in Increased Evaporation and Dry Eye Symptoms
Obstruction of the meibomian glands leads to decreased delivery of their oil onto the posterior lid margin that results in: (1) a thinning of the tear film lipid layer; (2) tear film instability; (3) increased evaporation [48] of the aqueous phase leading to an evaporative dry eye condition with consequent hyperosmolarity of the remaining tears [49]. Hyperosmolarity [24] exerts stress on the ocular surface epithelia (cornea and conjunctiva) that results in an activation of the cells [50] with the release of inflammatory mediators. This contributes to the well-known signs and symptoms of a dry eye condition – such as stinging, burning and foreign body sensation – together with vital staining of the epithelial surface due to mechanical alteration from increased friction between the lids and bulbus, and is associated with reduced and unstable visual acuity [36, 51–53]. Continued activation of the ocular surface epithelia can lead to the onset of a self-enforcing inflammatory cascade that is modulated via a deregulation of the physiological mucosal immune system of the ocular surface, the eye-associated lymphoid tissue [54–56], see another contribution to this volume). This may, in advanced chronic stages, require an immunomodulatory therapeutic intervention [1, 57, 58].

Anatomy and Pathology of the MCJ of the Lid Margin

Currently, the definition of the MCJ of the human lid margin is not very precise. This is reflected by descriptions that apparently regard the whole epithelial thickening (now identified as the lid wiper [59–61]) as the MCJ [35, 62], whereas others have defined the MCJ as only a narrow division line between the cornified epidermis and the conjunctiva [30]. These different descriptions reflect the fact that only scant knowledge exists about this structure.

Line of Marx Is the Surface of the MCJ

Historical investigations have reported that the MCJ lies on the posterior part of the free lid margin at the level of the posterior rim of the meibomian orifices where the skin epidermis stops [63]. By in vivo confocal laser scanning microscopy of individuals around the fourth decade of life [61], it was seen that the epidermis ends sharply in about the midline through the orifices of the meibomian glands, but at an orifice this is completely encircled by an epidermal cuff. This is also a typical finding in histology of individuals aged in their mid-seventies [61], although sometimes the posterior rim of the meibomian gland orifice can already be covered by a non-cornified parakeratinized epithelium. Age dependent anterior movement of the line of Marx [64] and posterior movement of the orifices of the meibomian glands (retroplacement) [28] are shown as typical findings in aging. After the abrupt stop of the epidermis the MCJ starts and represents the transition zone between skin and mucous membrane.

In the same position, Marx [16] described a line that he observed in great detail after the application of several types of vital stains; this line is therefore known as the 'line of Marx' (fig. 4). Before him, Virchow [38] had also mentioned an 'admarginal zone' that was characterized by the intense uptake of pikrin and eosin stains. Marx reported that stained dots accumulate on the posterior lid margin, and these represent single or groups of surface cells, which condense towards the outside (i.e. to the skin) into a homogeneous thin line [16]. These basic findings have been supported by other authors [17, 19]. The functional significance of this vital staining line has remained a subject of speculation. Marx noted that this line: (1) has a relation to the outer margin of the tear meniscus; (2) may be caused by the interaction of the tears with the epithelium; (3) may serve to guide the tears along the lid margin to the lacrimal punctum. Ehlers [19] suggested it might be caused by friction during blinking, while Norn observed that it represented the bottom of the tear meniscus which argues against a direct contact with the globe and respective mechanical forces in this region.

Recent histological investigations have shown that the epithelium that follows after the abrupt stop of the keratin layers of the cornified epidermis is still stratified squamous, but the cytoplasm of the surface cells is very dense and still contains a nucleus which characterizes them as parakeratinized [61]. These cells stained very intensely with Masson-Goldners trichrome stain, which contains red acidic fuchsine, one of the stains already used by Marx (fig. 4). The parakeratinized cells of this continuous zone later disperse into single parakeratinized cells among ordinary brighter squamous cells. The reported results using Masson-Goldners trichrome stain on histological sections perfectly matched what had been described by Marx in his vital staining procedure. Therefore, it can be concluded that this narrow zone of parakeratinized cells located at the surface of the MCJ represents the histological equivalent of the vital staining line of Marx and the line of Marx is hence the surface of the ocular MCJ. On the crest of the inner lid border, the MCJ transforms into epithelium with a conjunctival structure composed of roundish cells of less density. This epithelial cushion forms the lid wiper (fig. 5).

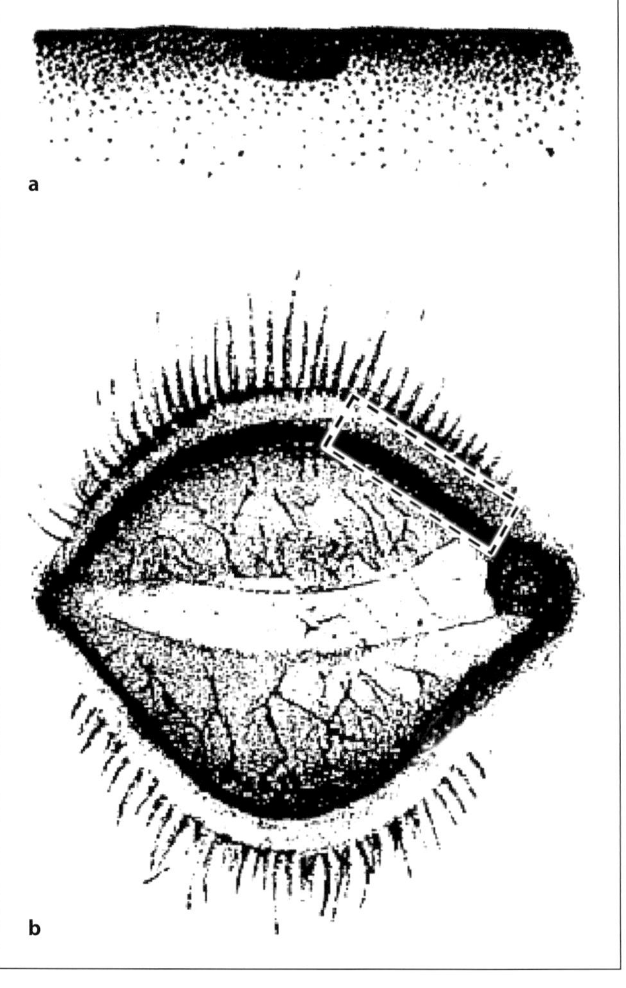

Fig. 4. Original drawing of the line of Marx. According to the original drawing by E. Marx, the vital staining line (dotted box in enlargement **a**) that he described in his paper in 1924 is located at the inner border of the eye lid 'between palpebral conjunctiva and lid margin' as indicated in **b**. It consists of single dots of vital-stained cells that increasingly accumulate from the conjunctival side (**a**, bottom) into a dense line towards the skin (**a**, top). The stained line also encircles the lacrimal punctum and extends into it, seen as a large dark spot in **a**. From Marx [16].

MCJ/Line of Marx Can Be Used as a Diagnostic Tool in Dry Eye Research

The line of Marx has meanwhile received increased interest because it can be easily stained (e.g. by the vital stains fluorescein, lissamine green and rose bengal) and its functional and pathological significance are under speculation [64, 65]. It was considered that this line may be the natural site of contact [65, 66] between the eyelid margin and the surfaces of the bulbus (conjunctiva and cornea). However, this appears to be unlikely due to several reasons: (1) as judged from the lid geometry, the line of Marx is too far outside, i.e. distal, on the posterior lid border to touch the globe – this is supported by the observation that it starts at the posterior margin of the meibomian gland orifices [17, 19, 64] and represents the bottom of the tear meniscus [17]; (2) this zone is too narrow; (3) it appears to be too rigid – as judged from its composition of parakeratinized cells [61] and compared to the conceivably soft cushion of the conjunctival

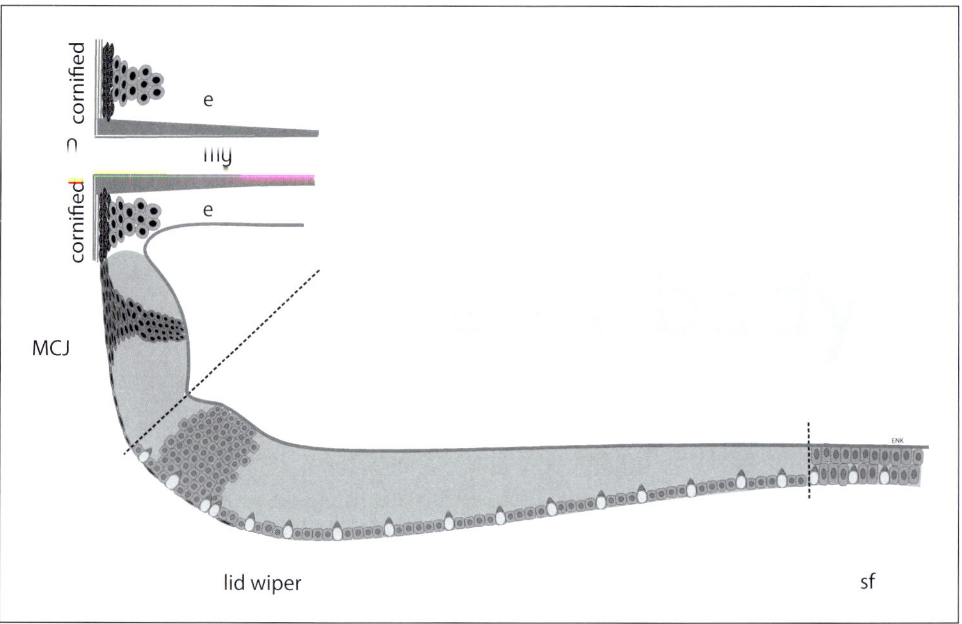

Fig. 5. Schematic drawing of the inner lid border including the meibomian gland orifice, MCJ and lid wiper, and related cell types. The different zones of the posterior lid border on the inside of the eyelid body consist of the opening (o) of the meibomian gland (mg), which is typically located still within the cornified epidermis (e). This is followed by the vital stainable 'line of Marx', which consists of flat parakeratinized surface cells and represents the surface of the MCJ. The MCJ ends at the crest of the inner lid border. At the crest (dotted line between MCJ and lid wiper), the stratified cubical epithelium of the lid wiper starts. It regularly contains goblet cells and varying numbers of flat and PK cells, continuing those that gradually disseminate from the line of Marx. The lid wiper forms an epithelial cushion and gradually decreases in thickness until it transforms into the epithelium of the subtarsal fold (sf).

structure of the more proximal lid wiper – to prevent destruction of the sensitive bulbar epithelia during the continuous travelling of the lid margin during the frequent physiological eye blinks.

The natural stainable line that occurs after application of vital stains was also assumed to indicate the functionality of the meibomian glands because these usually open in front (i.e. distal to it) on the free lid margin. This appears to have considerable clinical importance because meibomian oils are naturally delivered onto the tear meniscus [26] that starts around the posterior rim of the meibomian orifices and is located on the surface of the MCJ/line of Marx [17]. With increasing age, in blepharitis and in meibomian gland disease, however, the line of Marx moves in an anterior direction [64] and the orifices are also reported to move backwards (retroplacement) [28]. Both of these facts indicate a location of the orifice inside the tear meniscus, and consequently the delivery of meibomian oil into the tear meniscus rather than on top of it which conceivably results in an ineffective formation of the tear film lipid layer.

It is therefore not surprising that the location of the line of Marx was found to be strongly correlated with meibomian gland function. The observation of its location relative to the meibomian gland orifices is therefore suggested as a rapid and efficient clinical procedure at slit lamp examination for the assessment of meibomian gland function [64].

Anatomy and Pathology of the Lid Wiper

The MCJ on the posterior part of the free lid margin, behind the orifices of the meibomian glands, is followed on the crest of the inner lid border into the direction of the fornix by a stratified epithelium of a clearly conjunctival structure that represents the lid wiper (fig. 5). It contains cubical and even prismatic cells with a less dense cytoplasm and also, typically, goblet cells. This represents the start of the conjunctival mucosa, although some squamous and PK cells are still interspersed at the surface and continue those of the line of Marx, which again supports the original observations of Marx who reported that stained dots, recently verified as parakeratinized cells, fade out gradually to the conjunctival side.

The Lid Wiper Is the Device at the Inner Lid Border That Distributes the Thin Preocular Tear Film

The epithelium of this marginal conjunctival zone is stratified, has initially about 8–12 cell layers, and (further down to the proximal side in the direction of the fornix) the number of cell layers and the vertical height of the epithelium gradually decreases until it transforms into the epithelium of the subtarsal fold (fig. 5). This epithelium hence forms a thick cushion as judged by the cell shape and loose arrangement compared to the MCJ. The goblet cells, which are frequently arranged in groups, can provide a built-in lubrication system in order to decrease frictional forces between this epithelium and the bulbar surface, and further support that this is the zone which actually travels over the bulbar epithelium during every blink. Since this zone starts on the crest of the inner lid border and extends towards the tarsal side, it is also in a geometrically suitable location to be directly apposed to the globe, in contrast to the more distal zone of the line of Marx, i.e. the surface of the MCJ.

Due to its proposed function, this zone of the marginal conjunctiva is termed the 'lid wiper' [59, 60]. A thickening of the epithelium on the conjunctival side of the inner lid border was first reported by Virchow [38] and later by Ehlers [19]; the latter termed it a 'wind screen wiper' in analogy to the device of a car.

Lid Wiper Epitheliopathy Is a Sensitive Early Indicator of a Dry Eye

Even though this arrangement has immediate functional implications for the distribution of the tear film, until recently it had received limited attention. It gained interest when Korb et al. [60], who discovered pathological alterations in this area, termed

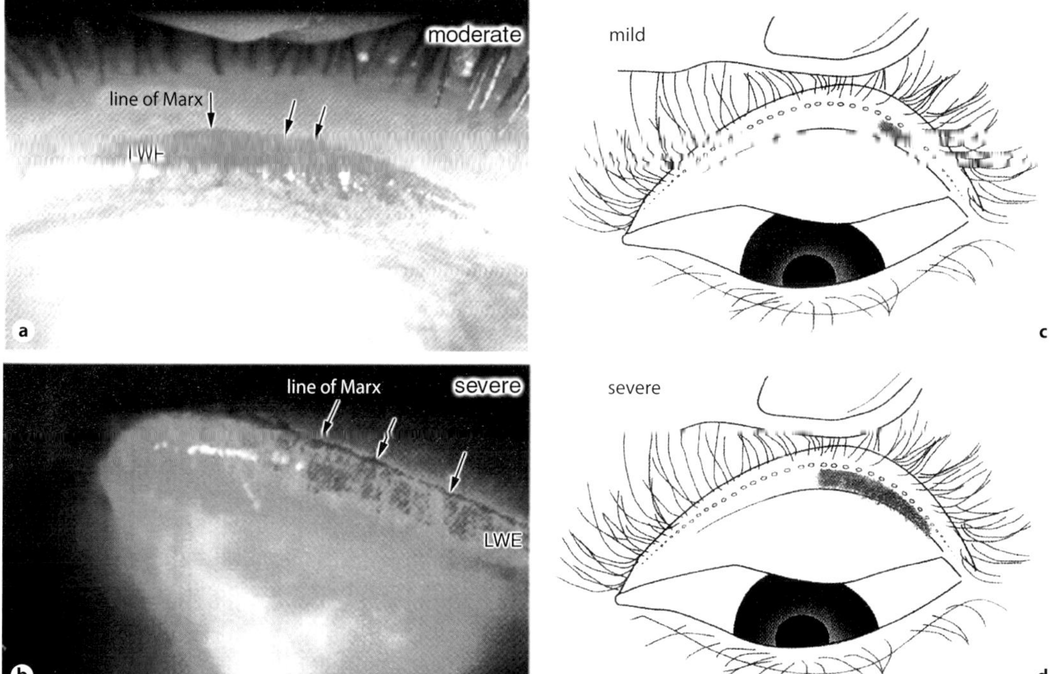

Fig. 6. Lid wiper epitheliopathy (LWE). In wetting deficiencies of contact lens wearers and in dry eye disease, the lid wiper is the first zone of the ocular surface that shows morphological alterations in the epithelium that are detectable in a vital staining, e.g. by rose bengal (**a**) or by fluorescein (**b**). LWE can be graded depending on the extension of staining (horizontal width along the lid margin and sagittal length proportional to the length of lid wiper zone) into mild (**c**), moderate (**a**) or severe stages (**b**, **d**) which reflects the severity of the wetting deficiency. Reproduced with permission from Korb et al. [59, 60].

it the 'lid wiper'; the pathological alterations in this zone were termed lid wiper epitheliopathy (LWE) [59, 60]. As shown in figure 6, LWE: (1) is an alteration in the epithelium of the portion of the marginal conjunctiva of the upper eyelid that wipes the ocular surface; (2) is diagnosed by vital staining; (3) is correlated to dry eye symptoms and disease [59, 60]; (4) occurs more frequently in patients with dry eye symptoms than in normal controls; (5) may be a sensitive early indicator of tear film instability and dry eye disease, as it may occur in either the presence or absence of conventional signs (Schirmer's test and tear film break-up time) [60].

Conclusion

In conclusion, the lid margin has an eminent and yet underestimated influence on the intact formation of the precorneal tear film, and hence also on the preservation of ocular surface integrity and visual function. Consequently, pathological alterations in the lid margin also have a large and equally underestimated impact on the onset and course of dry eye disease, which have only recently begun to be unraveled. Similar to dry eye disease at the ocular surface proper (conjunctiva and cornea), the pathology at the lid margin also has, if undiagnosed and untreated, a tendency to self-propagate and to aggravate in vicious circles [67]. This concerns in particular a degenerative atrophic destruction of the meibomian gland structure inside the eyelids, but also contributes to corneal and conjunctival pathology. It is therefore of importance that the lid margin receives increased attention by the clinician and that a thorough investigation of the lid margin should be part of every investigation of a patient via the slit lamp, and in particular of patients of older age, before contact lens fitting and of those with incipient, or more advanced, symptoms of dry eye disease.

Acknowledgments

Supported by Deutsche Forschungsgemeinschaft (DFG KN317/11)

References

1 Knop E, Knop N, Brewitt H: Dry eye disease as a complex dysregulation of the functional anatomy of the ocular surface. New impulses to understanding dry eye disease (in German). Ophthalmologe 2003;100:917–928.

2 Bron AJ, Tiffany JM: The contribution of meibomian disease to dry eye. Ocul Surf 2004;2:149–165.

3 Zierhut M, Dana MR, Stern ME, Sullivan DA: Immunology of the lacrimal gland and ocular tear film. Trends Immunol 2002;23:333–335.

4 King-Smith PE, Fink BA, Hill RM, Koelling KW, Tiffany JM: The thickness of the tear film. Curr Eye Res 2004;29:357–368.

5 Knop E, Knop N: New techniques in lacrimal gland research: the magic juice and how to drill for it. Opthalmic Res 2008;40:2–4.

6 Holly FJ: Tear film physiology. Am J Optom Physiol Opt 1980;57:252–257.

7 Rüfer F, Brewitt H: Das Trockene Auge. Klin Monatsbl Augenheilkd 2004;221:R51.-R70.

8 Heiligenhaus A, Koch JM, Kemper D, Kruse FE, Waubke TN: Therapy in tear film deficiencies (in German). Klin Monatsbl Augenheilkd 1994;204:162–168.

9 Shimazaki J, Sakata M, Tsubota K: Ocular surface changes and discomfort in patients with meibomian gland dysfunction. Arch Ophthalmol 1995;113:1266–1270.

10 Holly FJ, Lemp M: Wettability and wetting of corneal epithelium. Exp Eye Res 1971;11:239–250.

11 Argueso P, Gipson IK: Epithelial mucins of the ocular surface: structure, biosynthesis and function. Exp Eye Res 2001;73:281–289.

12 Jumblatt JE, Jumblatt MM: Detection and quantification of conjunctival mucins. Adv Exp Med Biol 1998;438:239–246.

13 Cope C, Dilly PN, Kaura R, Tiffany JM: Wettability of the corneal surface: a reappraisal. Curr Eye Res 1986;5:777–785.

14 Lemp M, Holly FJ, Shuzo I, Dohlman C: The precorneal tear film. 1. Factors in spreading and maintaining a continuous tear film over the corneal surface. Arch Ophthalmol 1970;83:89–94.

15 Holly FJ: Formation and rupture of the tear film. Exp Eye Res 1973;15:515–525.

16 Marx E: Über vitale Färbungen am Auge und an den Lidern. I. Über Anatomie, Physiologie und Pathologie des Augenlidrandes und der Tränenpunkte. Graefes Arch Clin Exp Ophthalmol 1924;114:465–482.

17 Norn MS: Vital staining of the canaliculus lacrimalis and the palpebral border (Marx' line). Acta Ophthalmol (Copenh) 1966;44:948–959.

18 Parsons JH: Pathology of the Eye. London, Holder and Stoughton, 1904, vol 1: Histology, pp 2, 31.

19 Ehlers N: The precorneal film: biomicroscipical, histological and chemical investigations. Acta Ophthalmol Suppl 1965;81:1–134.

20 Korb DR, Baron DF, Herman JP, Finnemore VM, Exford JM, Hermosa JL, Leahy CD, Glonek T, Greiner JV: Tear film lipid layer thickness as a function of blinking. Cornea 1994;13:354–359.

21 Lemp MA: Precorneal fluid and blinking. Int Ophthalmol Clin 1981;21:55–66.

22 Tsubota K, Nakamori K: Effects of ocular surface area and blink rate on tear dynamics. Arch Ophthalmol 1995;113:155–158.

23 Mishima S, Maurice D: The oily layer of the tear film and evaporation from the corneal surface. Exp Eye Res 1961;1:39–45.

24 Gilbard JP, Farris RL: Tear osmolarity and ocular surface disease in keratoconjunctivitis sicca. Arch Ophthalmol 1979;97:1642–1646.

25 Mathers WD, Shields WJ, Sachdev MS, Petroll WM, Jester JV: Meibomian gland dysfunction in chronic blepharitis. Cornea 1991;10:277–285.

26 Bron AJ, Tiffany JM, Gouveia SM, Yokoi N, Voon LW: Functional aspects of the tear film lipid layer. Exp Eye Res 2004;78:347–360.

27 McDonald JE: Surface phenomena of tear films. Trans Am Ophthalmol Soc 1968;66:905–939.

28 Hykin PG, Bron AJ: Age-related morphological changes in lid margin and meibomian gland anatomy. Cornea 1992;11:334–342.

29 Holbach LM: Diseases of the eyelid-conjunctival complex and corneal complications of lid disease. Curr Opin Ophthalmol 1995;6:39–43.

30 Foulks GN, Bron AJ: Meibomian gland dysfunction: a clinical scheme for description, diagnosis, classification, and grading. Ocul Surf 2003;1:107–126.

31 Di Pascuale MA, Espana EM, Liu DT, Kawakita T, Li W, Gao YY, Baradaran-Rafii A, Elizondo A, Raju VK, Tseng SC: Correlation of corneal complications with eyelid cicatricial pathologies in patients with Stevens-Johnson syndrome and toxic epidermal necrolysis syndrome. Ophthalmology 2005;112:904–912.

32 McCulley JP, Shine WE: Eyelid disorders: the meibomian gland, blepharitis, and contact lenses. Eye Contact Lens 2003;29:S93–S95.

33 Den S, Shimizu K, Ikeda T, Tsubota K, Shimmura S, Shimazaki J: Association between meibomian gland changes and aging, sex, or tear function. Cornea 2006;25:651–655.

34 Hirotani Y, Yokoi N, Komuro A, Kinoshita S: Age-related changes in the mucocutaneous junction and the conjunctivochalasis in the lower lid margins (in Japanese). Nippon Ganka Gakkai Zasshi 2003;107:363–368.

35 Wirtschafter JD, Ketcham JM, Weinstock RJ, Tabesh T, McLoon LK: Mucocutaneous junction as the major source of replacement palpebral conjunctival epithelial cells. Invest Ophthalmol Vis Sci 1999;40:3138–3146.

36 Korb DR, Henriquez AS: Meibomian gland dysfunction and contact lens intolerance. J Am Optom Assoc 1980;51:243–251.

37a Knop E, Knop N, Brewitt H, Pleyer U, Rieck P, Seitz B, Schirra F: Meibomian Glands. III. Meibomian gland dysfunction (MGD) – plaidoyer for a discrete disease entity and as an important cause of dry eye (in German). Ophthalmologe 2009;106:966–979.

37b Knop E, Knop N, Schirra F: Meibomian glands. Part II: Physiology, characteristics, distribution and function of meibomian oil (in German). Ophthalmologe 2009;106:884–892.

38 Virchow H: Mikroskopische Anatomie der äusseren Augenhaut und des Lidapparates; in Saemisch T (ed): Graefe-Saemisch Handbuch der gesamten Augenheilkunde. Leipzig, Verlag W. Engelmann, 1910, vol 1, p 431.

39 Wolff E. Anatomy of the Eye and Orbit. London, Lewis and Co., 1954.

40 Duke-Elder S, Wybar KC: The Anatomy of the Visual System. London, Henry Kimpton, 1961, pp 577.

41 Knop N, Knop E: Meibomian glands. I. Anatomy, embryology and histology of the meibomian glands (in German). Ophthalmologe 2009;106:872–883.

42 Nicolaides N, Kaitaranta JK, Rawdah TN, Macy JI, Boswell FM, Smith RE: meibomian gland studies: comparison of steer and human lipids. Invest Ophthalmol Vis Sci 1981;20:522–536.

43 Bron AJ, Tripathi DM, Tripathi BJ: Wolff's Anatomy of the Eye and Orbit. London, Chapman & Hall Medical, 1997, p 231.

44 Kozak I, Bron AJ, Kucharova K, Kluchova D, Marsala M, Heichel CW, Tiffany JM: Morphologic and volumetric studies of the meibomian glands in elderly human eyelids. Cornea 2007;26:610–614.

45 Knop E, Knop N, Zhivov A, Kraak R, Korb DR, Greiner JV, Guthoff R: Keratinisation and mucocutaneous junction of the human lid margin in relation to the meibomian gland orifice. Invest Ophthal Vis Sci 2009;50:4833.

46 Henriquez AS, Korb DR: Meibomian glands and contact lens wear. Br J Ophthalmol 1981;65:108–111.

47 Gutgesell VJ, Stern GA, Hood CI: Histopathology of meibomian gland dysfunction. Am J Ophthalmol 1982;94:383–387.

48 Mathers WD: Ocular evaporation in meibomian gland dysfunction and dry eye. Ophthalmology 1993;100:347–351.

49 Gilbard JP, Gray KL, Rossi SR: A proposed mechanism for increased tear-film osmolarity in contact lens wearers. Am J Ophthalmol 1986;102:505–507.

50 Luo L, Li DQ, Corrales RM, Pflugfelder SC: Hyperosmolar saline is a proinflammatory stress on the mouse ocular surface. Eye Contact Lens 2005;31:186–193.
51 Gilbard JP, Rossi SR, Gray KL: A new rabbit model for keratoconjunctivitis sicca. Invest Ophthalmol Vis Sci 1987;28:225–228.
52 McCulley JP, Sciallis GF: Meibomian keratoconjunctivitis. Am J Ophthalmol 1977;84:788–793.
53 Brewitt H, Kaercher T, Rüfer F: Dry eye and blepharitis (in German). Klin Monatsbl Augenheilkd 2008;225:R15–R36.
54 Knop E, Knop N: Eye-associated lymphoid tissue (EALT) is continuously spread throughout the ocular surface from the lacrimal gland to the lacrimal drainage system (in German). Ophthalmologe 2003; 100:929–942.
55 Knop E, Knop N: The role of eye-associated lymphoid tissue in corneal immune protection. J Anat 2005;206:271–285.
56 Knop E, Knop N: Conjunctiva immune surveillance; in Dartt DA, Edelhauser HF (eds): Encyclopedia of the Eye. Oxford, Elsevier, 2009.
57 Knop E, Knop N: Influence of the eye-associated lymphoid tissue (EALT) on inflammatory ocular surface disease. Ocul Surf 2005;3:S180–S186.
58 McDermott AM, Perez V, Huang AJ, Pflugfelder SC, Stern ME, Baudouin C, Beuerman RW, Burns AR, Calder VL, Calonge M, Chodosh J, Coster DJ, Dana R, Hazlett LD, Jones DB, Kim SK, Knop E, Li DQ, Mitchell BM, Niederkorn JY, Pearlman E, Wilhelmus KR, Kurie E: Pathways of corneal and ocular surface inflammation: a perspective from the Cullen symposium. Ocul Surf 2005;3:S131–S138.
59 Korb DR, Herman JP, Greiner JV, Scaffidi RC, Finnemore VM, Exford JM, Blackie CA, Douglass T: Lid wiper epitheliopathy and dry eye symptoms. Eye Contact Lens 2005;31:2–8.
60 Korb DR, Greiner JV, Herman JP, Hebert E, Finnemore VM, Exford JM, Glonek T, Olson MC: Lid-wiper epitheliopathy and dry-eye symptoms in contact lens wearers. CLAO J 2002;28:211–216.
61 Knop E, Knop N, Zhivov A, Kraak R, Korb D, Greiner JV, Guthoff R: Definition of different subzones, including the lid wiper, in the marginal human conjunctiva by histology and in vivo confocal microscopy. Invest Ophthalmol Vis Sci 2008;49:5299.
62 Wolfram-Gabel R, Sick H: Microvascularization of the mucocutaneous junction of the eyelid in fetuses and neonates. Surg Radiol Anat 2002;24:97–101.
63 Wolff E: The mucocutaneous junction of the lid margin and the distribution of the tear fluid. Trans Ophthalmol Soc UK 1946;66:291–308.
64 Yamaguchi M, Kutsuna M, Uno T, Zheng X, Kodama T, Ohashi Y: Marx line: fluorescein staining line on the inner lid as indicator of meibomian gland function. Am J Ophthalmol 2006;141:669–675.
65 Doughty MJ, Naase T, Donald C, Hamilton L, Button NF: Visualisation of 'Marx's line' along the marginal eyelid conjunctiva of human subjects with lissamine green dye. Ophthalmic Physiol Opt 2004;24:1–7.
66 Shaw AJ, Collins MJ, Davis BA, Carney LG: Eyelid pressure: inferences from corneal topographic changes. Cornea 2009;28:181–188.
67 Knop E, Knop N: Meibomian glands. IV. Functional interactions in the pathogenesis of meibomian gland Dysfunction (MGD). Ophthalmologe 2009; 106:980–987.

PD Dr. Erich Knop
Research Laboratory of the Department of Ophthalmology CVK, Charité – Universitätsmedizin Berlin
Ziegelstrasse 5–9
DE–10117 Berlin (Germany)
E-Mail erich.knop@charite.de

Brewitt H (ed): Research Projects in Dry Eye Syndrome.
Dev Ophthalmol. Basel, Karger, 2010, vol 45, pp 123–128

Diagnostic Markers of Sjögren's Syndrome

Torsten Witte

Klinik für Immunologie und Rheumatologie, Medizinische Hochschule Hannover, Hannover, Germany

Abstract

Establishing a diagnosis of Sjögren's syndrome (SS) has been difficult without sensitive laboratory markers, and in light of the non-specificity of the symptoms of dry eyes and mouth. Rather than complaints about dry eyes or dry mouth, objective symptoms and extraglandular manifestations should raise suspicion of SS. This evaluation requires the detection of antibodies against Ro (SSA) and La (SSB) or a pathologic salivary gland biopsy. Since an invasive biopsy is not always performed, further diagnostic markers are required. Recently antibodies against α-fodrin have been shown to be present in the majority of untreated patients, and can be used in the screening process of SS as an additional marker.

Sjögren's syndrome (SS) is an autoimmune disease characterized by lymphocytic infiltration into the lachrymal and salivary glands, leading to dry eyes and mouth. The infiltration may also occur in extraglandular sites, such as the kidneys, lungs and liver. Most infiltrating lymphocytes are CD4+ T cells. SS is a major cause of dry eyes and mouth and affects up to 0.5% of the population. In the USA, SS patients are estimated to generate an annual healthcare cost of USD 10.3 billion (only surpassed by rheumatoid arthritis) [1].

Current Diagnostic Procedures in SS

Although SS is common, it is difficult to diagnose since objective reductions in tear and saliva production are frequent. These may be caused by infections (hepatitis C, HIV), sarcoidosis or drugs (diuretics, tricyclic antidepressants, β-blockers), and are often observed in elderly people. In addition, only a minority of the individuals with reduced tear and saliva production complain of subjective symptoms. In contrast, patients with depression often complain of dry eyes and mouth even in the presence of normal glandular function. Even though questions to detect dry eyes and dry mouth have been developed (table 1) [2], they were found to correlate only weakly or

Table 1. Symptoms of dry eyes and mouth suggested by the European Study Group of Sjögren's Syndrome [2]

Ocular Symptoms
1. Have you had daily, persistent, troublesome dry eyes for more than 3 months?
2. Do you have a recurrent sensation of sand or gravel in the eyes?
3. Do you use tear substitutes more than three times a day?
Oral Symptoms
1. Have you had a daily feeling of dry mouth for more than 3 months?
2. Have you had recurrently or persistently swollen salivary glands as an adult?
3. Do you frequently drink liquids to aid in swallowing dry food?

Table 2. Symptoms that should raise suspicion of dry eyes or mouth

Cornea ulcerations
Recurrent conjunctivitis
Intolerance of contact lenses
Problems in prolonged talking
Intolerance of spicy food
Oral candidiasis
Severe caries
Severe gingivitis

not at all with the objective test results of sicca syndrome in the general population [3]. Symptoms that should raise the clinician's suspicion of dry eyes and mouth are summarized in table 2, with further symptoms that should raise the suspicion of SS in table 3.

Due to the low specificity of complaints of dry eyes and mouth, an objective reduction in tear and saliva flow always has to be confirmed by appropriate tests, such as Schirmer's test for dry eyes and Saxon's test for dry mouth. When dry eyes and mouth are present, according to the current European/American consensus criteria of SS [4], the autoimmune disorder of SS has to be diagnosed either by a pathologic salivary gland biopsy or by the presence of autoantibodies against Ro (SSA) and/or La (SSB). Although SS clearly is associated with antibodies against Ro (SSA), the prevalence of

Table 3. Symptoms and laboratory abnormalities that should raise suspicion of SS

Palpable purpura
Raynaud's syndrome
Oligo-/polyarthritis
Polyneuropathy
Fever of unknown origin
Pulmonary fibrosis
Parotidomegaly
Mother of a child with congenital heart block or neonatal lupus
Elevated erythrocyte sedimentation rate
Hypergammaglobulinemia
Mixed cryoglobulinemia
Antinuclear antibodies and rheumatoid factors

these antibodies is only approximately 50% [5]. Patients with SS lacking this marker can only be diagnosed by a salivary gland biopsy, which is invasive and not always performed.

Therefore, further diagnostic markers of SS are needed. Recently, autoantibodies against α-fodrin have been discussed as an additional biomarker of SS.

Function of α-Fodrin

α-Fodrin is a widely expressed intracellular 240-kDa protein forming a heterodimer with β-fodrin, a 235-kDa molecule homologous to α-fodrin. The heterodimers are anchored to the plasma membrane and bind to actin, calmodulin and microtubules. The complex of actin and α-fodrin is involved in the process of secretion.

In apoptosis, which may be induced by chronic viral infections, α-fodrin is cleaved by caspase 3 into smaller fragments of 150 and 120 kDa. Both fragments have been detected in the salivary glands of patients with SS in substantial amounts [6]. The immune system is not tolerant to the cleavage products, and antibodies are generated when the α-fodrin fragments are persistently present.

In 1997, antibodies against α-fodrin were first described in a murine model of SS [7]. The development of these antibodies, and of SS, could be prevented by treatment with caspase inhibitors as well as by injection of α-fodrin before thymectomy. On the other hand, the injection of apoptotic cleavage products of α-fodrin induced autoantibodies, T cell stimulation and lymphocytic infiltration of salivary glands in normal mice. Thus, there is strong evidence for a crucial role of antibodies against α-fodrin in murine models of SS.

Prevalence of Antibodies against α-Fodrin in SS

In the first studies on patients with SS from Japan, the prevalence of IgG antibodies against α-fodrin detected by immunoblot analysis was 67–92%. In more recent studies, with larger fragments of α-fodrin (including the 150-kDa cleavage product) as antigens, the prevalence of IgG antibodies against α-fodrin in American patients with SS criteria was even 98% [8].

In our own observations using an ELISA assay, the prevalence of both IgG and IgA antibodies against α-fodrin was determined in SS using the revised European criteria, the American/European consensus criteria [4] and the highly stringent San Diego criteria [9] for classification of SS.

IgA antibodies against α-fodrin were more prevalent than IgG autoantibodies and were present in 88%, IgG antibodies against α-fodrin in 64%, and IgA and/or IgG antibodies against α-fodrin in 93% of the patients classified according to San Diego criteria [10]. The prevalence was lower in patients classified according to both the European Study Group and American/European consensus criteria. IgA antibodies against α-fodrin were present in 64% and IgG antibodies against α-fodrin in 50% of the patients.

In other studies however, the prevalence of antibodies against α-fodrin in SS was only 30–50%. The concentration of α-fodrin antibodies is reduced by immunosuppressive treatment and is higher in the early phase of the disease. In order to study the association of α-fodrin antibodies with sicca symptoms in the general (and therefore untreated) population, we examined participants at a summer festival of our medical school. All the 168 volunteers were asked for subjective symptoms of dry eyes and mouth; afterwards, the saliva and tear production were measured and blood was drawn for measuring autoantibodies. We detected both dry eyes and mouth in 4 participants. Three of those four individuals had IgA antibodies against α-fodrin, and none had antibodies against Ro or La [11]. Although a salivary gland biopsy was not performed in those patients and SS could not be definitely confirmed, the study suggests that antibodies against α-fodrin may be a sensitive marker of SS in the general population.

Specificity of Antibodies against α-Fodrin

We have detected IgA and IgG antibodies against α-fodrin in approximately 10–20% of patients with multiple sclerosis, but also in 20% of patients with rheumatoid arthritis and systemic lupus erythematosus (even in the absence of secondary SS), but only in 2% of blood donors [12].

Due to the high prevalence of α-fodrin antibodies in other inflammatory diseases, their main indication is not the differential diagnosis of connective tissue diseases. They are however helpful in the detection of SS in patients with possible extraglandular manifestations, such as polyneuropathy or CNS involvement.

Antibodies against α-Fodrin Are Activity Markers of SS

The concentration of IgA and IgG antibodies against α-fodrin correlated with the degree of lymphocytic infiltration in the salivary glands, the erythrocyte sedimentation rate and hypergammaglobulinemia [13]. In several studies, antibodies against α-fodrin correlated with a shorter duration of SS and appeared before Ro antibodies [14].

In a recent retrospective evaluation, we could demonstrate that hydroxychloroquine treatment of SS patients significantly improves saliva production only in SS patients with (but not without) antibodies against α-fodrin [15]. Antibodies against α-fodrin may indicate early active disease, which is still treatable by immunosuppression. In agreement, rituximab treatment was recently shown to improve the saliva production only in SS patients with early disease [16]. Therefore, even though immunosuppressants have been regarded as ineffective in improving the glandular function in SS, there appears to be a therapeutic 'window of opportunity' which is indicated by the presence of α-fodrin antibodies.

Outlook

In order to further increase the sensitivity and specificity of antibodies against α-fodrin for SS, we are currently localizing their exact epitopes on the large protein. In previous studies, these epitopes have been roughly mapped in the N-terminal domain of α-fodrin in SS, but in a different domain in systemic lupus erythematosus [17]. The usage of these epitopes instead of the whole protein as an antigen in ELISA tests could make the autoantibodies an even more specific marker of SS, which should be determined in addition to antibodies against Ro/La.

References

1 Shoenfeld Y, Selmi C, Zimlichman E, Gershwin ME: The autoimmunologist: geoepidemiology, a new center of gravity and prime time for autoimmunity. J Autoimmun 2008;31:325–330.

2 Vitali C, Bombardieri S, Moutsopoulos HM, Balestrieri G, Bencivelli W, Bernstein RM, Bjerrum KB, Braga S, Coll J, de Vita S, et al: Preliminary criteria for the classification of Sjögren's syndrome: results of a prospective concerted action supported by the European Community. Arthritis Rheum 1993;6:340–347.

3 Hay EM, Thomas E, Pal B, Hajeer A, Chambers H, Silman AJ: Weak association between subjective symptoms or and objective testing for dry eyes and dry mouth: results from a population based study. Ann Rheum Dis 1998;57:20–24.

4 Vitali C, Bombardieri S, Jonsson R, Moutsopoulos HM, Alexander EL, Carsons SE, Daniels TE, Fox PC, Fox RI, Kassan SS, Pillemer SR, Talal N, Weisman MH: European Study Group on Classification Criteria for Sjogren's Syndrome. Classification criteria for Sjögren's syndrome: a revised version of the European criteria proposed by the American-European Consensus Group. Ann Rheum Dis 2002;61:554–558.

5 Ramos-Casals M, Solans R, Rosas J, Camps MT, Gil A, Del Pino-Montes J, Calvo-Alen J, Jiménez-Alonso J, Micó ML, Beltrán J, Belenguer R, Pallarés L, GEMESS Study Group: Primary Sjögren syndrome in Spain: clinical and immunologic expression in 1010 patients. Medicine 2008;87:210–219.

6 Martin SJ, O'Brien GA, Nishioka WK, McGahon AJ, Mahboubi A, Saido TC, Green DR: Proteolysis of fodrin (non-erythroid spectrin) during apoptosis. J Biol Chem 1995;270:6425–6428.

7 Haneji N, Nakamura T, Takio K, Yanagi K, Higashiyama H, Saito I, Noji S, Sugino H, Hayashi Y: Identification of alpha-fodrin as a candidate autoantigen in primary Sjögren's syndrome. Science 1997;276:604–607.

8 Maruyama T, Saito I, Hayashi Y, Kompfner E, Fox RI, Burton DR, Ditzel HJ: Molecular analysis of the human autoantibody response to alpha-fodrin in Sjögren's syndrome reveals novel apoptosis-induced specificity. Am J Pathol 2004;165:53–61.

9 Fox RI, Robinson C, Curd JC, Michelson P, Kozin F Howell FV: Sjögren's syndrome: proposed criteria for classification. Arthritis Rheum 1986;29:577–585.

10 Witte T, Matthias T, Oppermann M, Helmke K, Peter HH, Schmidt RE, Tishler M: Prevalence of antibodies against alpha-fodrin in Sjögren's syndrome: comparison of two sets of classification criteria. J Rheumatol 2003;30:2157–2159.

11 Witte T, Bierwirth J, Schmidt RE, Matthias T: Antibodies against alpha-fodrin are associated with dry eyes and mouth in the general population. J Rheumatol 2006;33:1713.

12 De Seze J, Dubucquoi S, Fauchais AL, Matthias T, Devos D, Castelnovo G, Stojkovic T, Ferriby D, Hachulla E, Labauge P, Lefranc D, Hatron PY, Vermersch P, Witte T: alpha-Fodrin autoantibodies in the differential diagnosis of MS and Sjogren syndrome. Neurology 2003;61:268–269.

13 Willeke P, Gaubitz M, Schotte H, Becker H, Mickholz E, Domschke W, Schlüter B: Clinical and immunological characteristics of patients with Sjögren's syndrome in relation to alpha fodrin antibodies. Rheumatology 2007;46:479–483.

14 Kobayashi I, Kawamura N, Okano M, Shikano T, Mizumoto M, Hayashi Y, Kobayashi K: Anti-alpha-fodrin autoantibody is an early diagnostic marker for childhood primary Sjögren's syndrome. J Rheumatol 2001;28:363–365.

15 Rihl M, Ulbricht K, Schmidt RE, Witte T: Treatment of sicca symptoms with hydroxychloroquine in patients with Sjogren's syndrome. Rheumatology 2009;48:796–799.

16 Pijpe J, van Imhoff GW, Vissink A, van der Wal JE, Kluin PM, Spijkervet FK, Kallenberg CG, Bootsma H: Changes in salivary gland immunohistology and function after rituximab monotherapy in a patient with Sjogren's syndrome and associated MALT lymphoma. Ann Rheum Dis 2005;64:958–960.

17 Chen Q, Li X, He W, Zhang H, Gao A, Cheng Y, Lei J, Li S, Zeng L: The epitope study of alpha-fodrin autoantibody in primary Sjögren's syndrome. Clin Exp Immunol 2007;149:497–503.

Prof. Dr. Torsten Witte
Klinik für Immunologie und Rheumatologie, Medizinische Hochschule Hannover
Carl-Neuberg-Strasse 1
DE–30625 Hannover (Germany)
Tel. +49 511 532 3014, Fax +49 511 532 5648, E-Mail witte.torsten@mh-hannover.de

Brewitt H (ed): Research Projects in Dry Eye Syndrome.
Dev Ophthalmol. Basel, Karger, 2010, vol 45, pp 129–138

Hyperosmolarity of the Tear Film in Dry Eye Syndrome

Elisabeth M. Messmer · Meral Bulgen · Anselm Kampik

Department of Ophthalmology, Ludwig Maximilian University, Munich, Germany

Abstract

Hyperosmolarity of the tear film is recognized as an important pathogenetic factor in dry eye syndrome (DES). Hyperosmolarity testing has been hampered in the past by difficulties in tear collection and analytic procedures that required laboratory facilities. The Tearlab™ Osmolarity System is a new user-friendly tool that only needs tiny volumes for analysis and determines hyperosmolarity semiautomatically. We measured tear film osmolarity with the Tearlab in 200 healthy individuals and patients with DES. Dry eye diagnosis was established when ≥3 of the following criteria were fulfilled: (1) Ocular Surface Disease Index >15; (2) staining of the cornea in the typical interpalpebral area; (3) staining of the conjunctiva in the typical interpalpebral area; (4) tear film break-up time <7 s; (5) Schirmer test <7 mm in 5 min; (6) the presence of blepharitis or meibomitis. Tear film osmolarity, as measured by Tearlab, did not show any correlation with the 6 clinical signs of dry eye. Moreover, tear film osmolarity testing could not discriminate between patients with DES (308.9 ± 14.0 mosm/l) and the control group (307.1 ± 11.3 mosml/l). Tear film osmolarity did not correlate to artificial tear use. Technical problems with the Tearlab, reflex tearing, or the difficulty in establishing a dry eye diagnosis with the recommended tests may account for these results. Further investigations are necessary before recommending this tool for daily clinical practice.

In 1941, von Bahr [1] postulated an association of tear film osmolarity with tear production and evaporation. Balik [2], in 1952, was the first to propose that hyperosmolarity of the tear film was a pathogenetic factor in dry eye syndrome (DES). The recent definition of DES published by the Dry Eye Workshop in 2007 supports this hypothesis and explicitly mentioned hyperosmolarity as a central finding in DES. Moreover, it established hyperosmolarity as one of the major pathogenetic mechanisms in dry eye [3].

Hyperosmolarity of the tear film stimulates a cascade of inflammatory events in corneal and conjunctival epithelial cells. Activation of protein kinases (MAP kinases) and nuclear transcription factors causes the production of proinflammatory cytokines, such as IL-1α, IL-1β, TNF-α, IL-8 and metalloproteinases (MMP-1, 3, 9 and

13) [4–6]. A subsequent inflammatory response results in apoptosis of conjunctival, corneal and lacrimal gland epithelia, keratinization and neuronal damage [4, 6–10]. Hyperosmolarity of the tear film significantly correlates with rose bengal staining of the ocular surface and the use of artificial tears [11, 12]. It is inversely proportional to tear production, as measured by Schirmer test with anesthesia [11].

Osmolarity of the normal tear film is 302 ± 6.3 mosm/l [13, 14]. In DES, tear film osmolarity increases up to 340 mosm/l [14] and is most pronounced in patients with combined aqueous deficiency and evaporative dry eye [15].

Some authors feel that tear film osmolarity testing is the most important diagnostic tool in the diagnosis of DES [16]. Tear film osmolarity as a single test was superior to lactate measurements, Schirmer testing and bengal rose staining of the ocular surface in a study by Tomlinson et al. [16]. Unfortunately, measurement of tear film osmolarity was mainly confined to laboratory settings using osmometers, which analyze colligative properties (such as freezing-point depression, vapor pressure or boiling-point elevation).

Only few months ago, a user-friendly osmometer came to the market (Tearlab™ Osmolarity System, OcuSense, Los Angeles, Calif., USA). In contrast to older osmometers, this tool only needs tiny tear volumes for analysis. Osmolarity is determined semi-automatically.

We examined tear film osmolarity of 200 healthy individuals and patients with DES using the Tearlab osmometer in order to evaluate its potential in differentiating between patients with and without dry eye.

Patients and Methods

Tearlab Osmolarity System

The Tearlab Osmolarity System requires less than 50 nl of tear fluid for analysis. After calibration of the instrument, tears are collected directly from the eye, eliminating the need for a standard glass capillary tube. Embedded nanofluidic channels move the tear sample to the measuring electrodes. Sampling time is reduced to less than 1 s. At the core of the Tearlab is a disposable lab-on-a-chip system that functions as both a tear collection device and a measurement system (fig. 1). A desktop instrument converts the electrical signals generated from the lab card into a quantitative measurement and displays it to the user. The cutoff value provided by the company is 316 mosm/l. The entire workflow, from sample to result, requires less than 2 min.

Patients

Two hundred healthy volunteers and patients with DES were included in this study.

Dry eye symptoms were documented with the Ocular Surface Disease Index (OSDI) questionnaire, and artificial tear use was recorded. Thereafter, patients underwent visual acuity testing and a thorough slit lamp examination. Before any additional tests, Tearlab osmolarity was analyzed in the subjectively worse eye or the left eye. Subsequently, lissamine staining of the

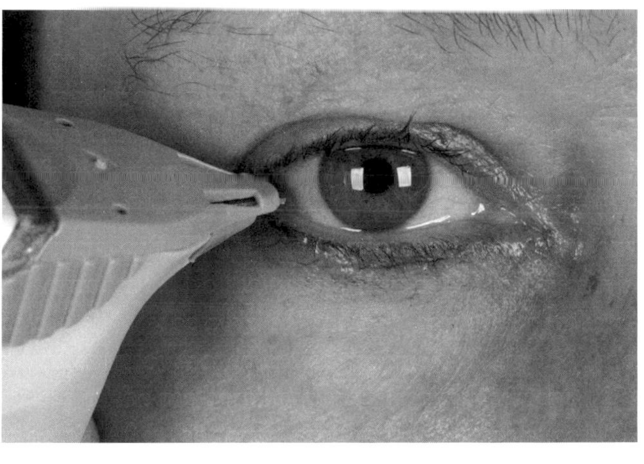

Fig. 1. Tearlab chip that that functions as a tear collection device and a measurement system.

conjunctiva, fluorescein staining of the cornea, break-up time and Schirmer test with and without anesthesia were performed. Corneal and conjunctival staining were evaluated using the Oxford Scheme [23]. The lowest Schirmer test value was used for analysis. Special attention was paid to the presence/absence of blepharitis and/or meibomitis.

An OSDI score >15, any staining of the cornea and/or conjunctiva in the typical interpalpebral area, a break-up time <7 s, a Schirmer test <7 mm in 5 min, and the presence of blepharitis/meibomitis was judged as a dry eye sign. When ≥3 of 6 dry eye signs were present, the patient was recruited into the DES group. Subjects with <3 dry eye signs/symptoms were assumed to have no clinically relevant DES.

Statistical analyses were performed using Pearson and Spearman correlations, as well as Wilcoxon and Mann-Whitney U tests.

Results

Only 16 of 200 patients showed no signs and/or symptoms of DES. In 71 patients, up to 2 signs/symptoms of DES were obvious. These individuals constitute the control group. On the other hand, 129 patients suffered from 3–6 dry eye signs/symptoms and were recruited into the DES group. Only 8 patients showed all 6 dry eye signs and symptoms (table 1). Median ages were 39 years (16–83) and 55 years (19–86) in the control and DES groups, respectively. In the DES group, 81 of 129 patients (62.8%), and in the control group 44 of 71 individuals (62.0%), were female.

Correlation of Tear Film Osmolarity with Age

Tear film osmolarity correlated significantly with the age of the patient ($p = 0.007$; fig. 2). However, when analyzing osmolarity values in the various age groups, no clear rise in osmolarity with increasing age was evident.

Table 1. Number of dry eye signs and symptoms in the study group

DES signs or symptoms, n	Patients, n
0	16
1	29
2	26
3	44
4	46
5	31
6	8

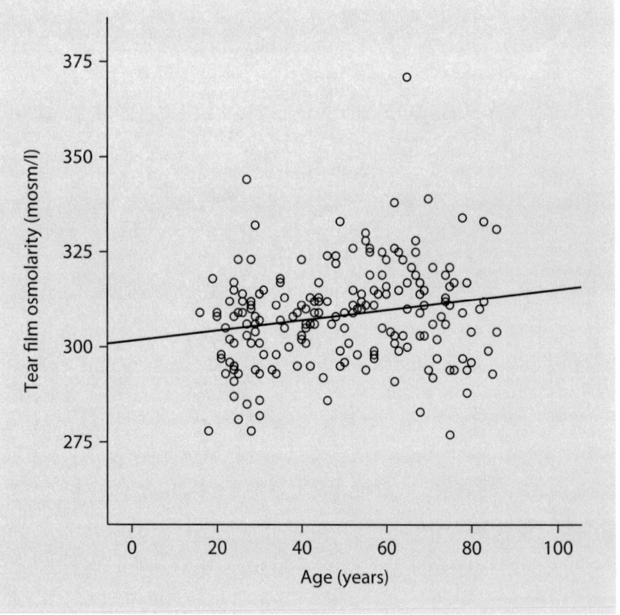

Fig. 2. Correlation of tear film osmolarity with age. A statistically significant correlation was obvious ($p = 0.007$).

Correlation of Tear Film Osmolarity to Single Signs of DES

Tear film osmolarity was correlated to all 6 signs of dry eye. No correlation of Tearlab osmolarity was seen with subjective symptoms of DES, as documented by the OSDI questionnaire (fig. 3), break-up time, Schirmer test values (fig. 4), the presence or absence of corneal/conjunctival staining, and blepharitis. Moreover, tear film

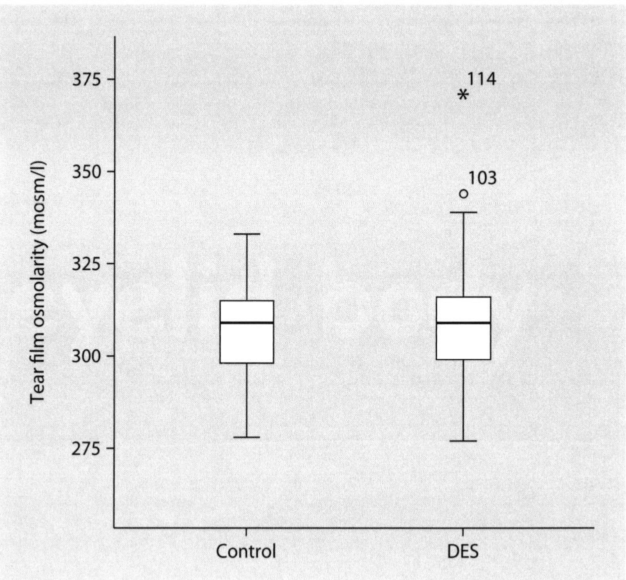

Fig. 3. Correlation of tear film osmolarity with dry eye symptoms as documented by OSDI. No correlation was evident.

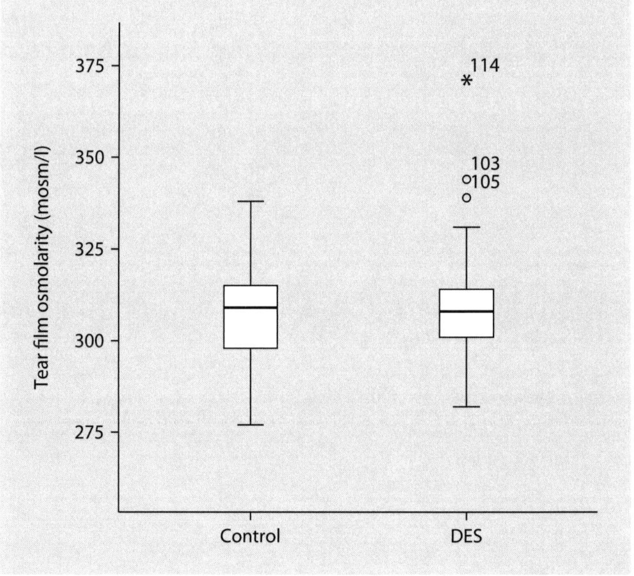

Fig. 4. Correlation of tear film osmolarity with Schirmer test. No correlation was detected.

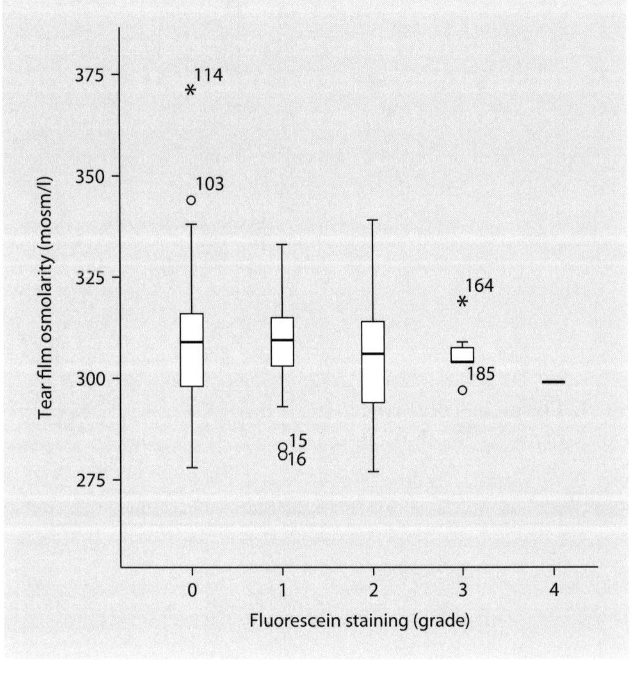

Fig. 5. Correlation of tear film osmolarity with fluorescein staining grades 0–4.

osmolarity as analyzed by Tearlab did not correspond to the degree of fluorescein staining (grades 1–4) (fig. 5) and lissamine staining (grades 1–3).

Correlation of Tear Film Osmolarity to Diagnosis of DES

Tear film osmolarities were 307.1 (SD 11.3) and 308.9 mosm/l (SD 14.0) in normal individuals and patients with DES, respectively. Tear film osmolarity in dry eye patients did not differ significantly from values obtained in the control group, even when ≥5 of 6 dry eye signs/symptoms were present and patients were clinically perceived as severe DES patients (fig. 6).

Moreover, tear film osmolarity did not correspond to the use of artificial tears (fig. 7).

Discussion

Tear film osmolarity testing is thought to be a useful parameter in dry eye diagnosis. Some authors even propagate introducing tear film osmolarity as the gold standard. If a cutoff value of 311 mosm/l is used, a single measurement of tear film osmolarity would reach a sensitivity of 59–95% with a specificity of 84–94% and a predictive

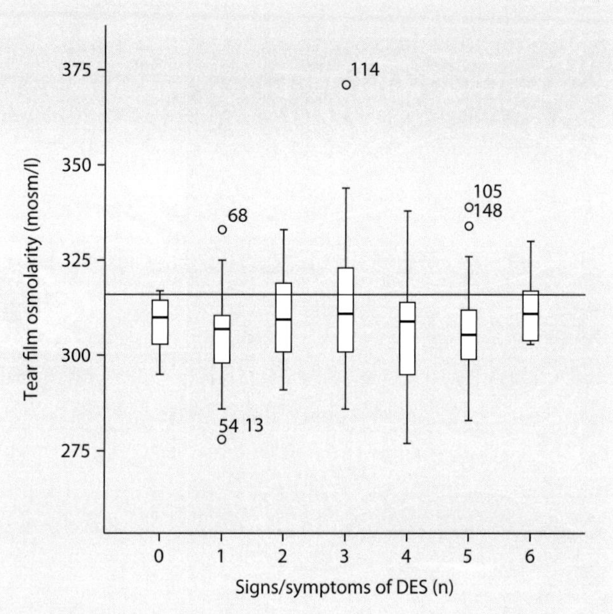

Fig. 6. Correlation of tear film osmolarity with DES characterized by increasing signs/symptoms of dry eye. An increase in tear film osmolarity was not even seen in patients with severe dry eye demonstrating ≥5 dry eye signs.

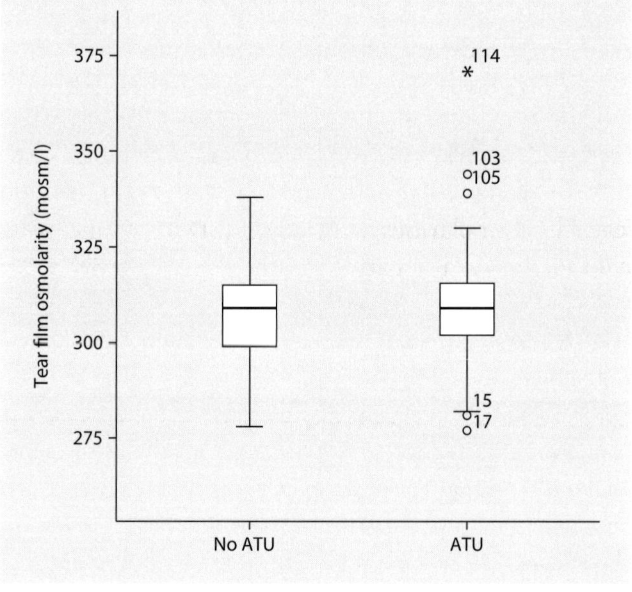

Fig. 7. Correlation of tear film osmolarity with artificial tear use (ATU). No correlation was evident.

value to diagnose 'dry eye' in 89% of published studies [13, 14, 16]. However, a significant overlap of values occurred between 293 and 320 mosml/l [16].

In our hands, tear film osmolarity testing using the recently available Tearlab Osmolarity System could not discriminate between healthy volunteers and patients with DES. A number of reasons may account for these results.

Tearlab Does Not Measure What It Is Supposed to Measure

The exact measurement principle of Tearlab is not publically available, nor could it be ascertained by direct enquiry to the company. Moreover, it is unknown whether the Tearlab measures osmolarity directly or indirectly (e.g. by determining salinity). In test solutions used for the calibration process for the instrument before use, however, meaningful results are obtained. Unfortunately, no studies analyzing tear film osmolarities with the Tearlab osmolarity system were available before introduction of the tool into the market.

We Measured the Wrong Area

In normal individuals, tear film osmolarity is supposed to be around 300 mosm/l. In dry eye patients, tear film osmolarity (as measured in the tear meniscus) only increases by approximately 50 mosm/l to reach 343 ± 32 mosm/l [14]. However, there are immense differences in tear film osmolarities between the tear meniscus and the bulbar tear film. Liu et al. [17] postulated osmolarity spikes of 800–900 mosm/l in areas of tear film break-up in DES. It may be difficult to measure small changes in tear film osmolarity in the tear meniscus by this technique. Thus, osmometry directly at the ocular surface may be a better technique for diagnosing DES.

We Measured Reflex Tears

Pathological changes can only be analyzed in basal tears, not in reflex tears [2, 14, 18]. The collection of tears is, therefore, critical for the measurement of meaningful osmolarities. Using filter papers or pipettes induces major reflex tearing by contact with conjunctiva and lids. In dry eye patients, harvesting of tears is even more difficult as tear volumes are significantly decreased [19]. The Tearlab chip is supposed to collect only minimal tear volumes directly from the tear film meniscus without inducing reflex tearing.

In our hands, medium tear film osmolarities in normal individuals and in DES patients were all below the given cutoff value of 316 mosm/l. It therefore seems quite possible that we did not obtain basal tears, but reflex tears with reduced osmolarity in our patients. As instructed in the operating manual, we tried to collect tears only from the temporal tear meniscus; however, touching the conjunctiva slightly was inevitable in most cases. Nevertheless, if measurements are distorted by such minimal alterations in harvesting tears, the Tearlab Osmolarity System is not ready for use in daily clinical practice.

Clinical Dry Eye Signs/Symptoms Used in This Study Are Not Able to Establish the Diagnosis of DES

The report of the International Dry Eye Workshop [3] recommends utilizing a clinical history, dry eye questionnaires, fluorescein break-up time, ocular surface staining, Schirmer testing, lid/meibomian morphology, and meibomian expression as practical tests for dry eye diagnosis. These tests were also applied in our study. Surprisingly, only 16 of 200 subjects showed no single feature of DES; 55 patients showed 1 or 2 signs/symptoms of dry eye, but were finally grouped into the control group according to other study protocols. Therefore, the discrimination between health and disease is not as clear as desirable. This could be a further reason for the missing correlation of tear film osmolarity with the diagnosis of DES. A weighting of specific dry eye signs and symptoms may be necessary to obtain better results. However, patients demonstrating all 6 dry eye signs and showing clinically severe DES did not show increased tear film osmolarity as compared to normal individuals in our study.

In conclusion, tear film osmolarity as measured by the Tearlab osmolarity system did not discriminate between our healthy volunteers and patients with DES. Further analysis is definitely necessary before recommending this instrument to the general ophthalmologist.

References

1 Von Bahr G: Könnte der Flüssigkeitsabgang durch die Cornea von physiologischer Bedeutung sein? Acta Ophthalmol 1941;19:125–134.
2 Balik J: The lacrimal fluid in keratoconjunctivitis sicca; a quantitative and qualitative investigation. Am J Ophthalmol 1952;35:1773–1782.
3 The definition and classification of dry eye disease: report of the Definition and Classification Subcommittee of the International Dry Eye WorkShop (2007). Ocul Surf 2007;5:75–92.
4 Li DQ, Chen Z, Song XJ, Luo L, Pflugfelder SC: Stimulation of matrix metalloproteinases by hyperosmolarity via a JNK pathway in human corneal epithelial cells. Invest Ophthalmol Vis Sci 2004; 45:4302–4311.
5 Li DQ, Luo L, Chen Z, Kim HS, Song XJ, Pflugfelder SC: JNK and ERK MAP kinases mediate induction of IL-1beta, TNF-alpha and IL-8 following hyperosmolar stress in human limbal epithelial cells. Exp Eye Res 2006;82:588–596.
6 Luo L, Li DQ, Corrales RM, Pflugfelder SC: Hyperosmolar saline is a proinflammatory stress on the mouse ocular surface. Eye Contact Lens 2005; 31:186–193.
7 Chen Z, Tong L, Li Z, Yoon KC, Qi H, Farley W, Li DQ, Pflugfelder SC : Hyperosmolarity-induced cornification of human corneal epithelial cells is regulated by JNK MAPK. Invest Ophthalmol Vis Sci 2008;49:539–549.

8 Luo L, Li DQ, Doshi A, Farley W, Corrales RM, Pflugfelder SC: Experimental dry eye stimulates production of inflammatory cytokines and MMP-9 and activates MAPK signaling pathways on the ocular surface. Invest Ophthalmol Vis Sci 2004;45:4293–4301.

9 Pflugfelder SC, de Paiva CS, Tong L, Luo L, Stern ME, Li DQ: Stress-activated protein kinase signaling pathways in dry eye and ocular surface disease. Ocul Surf 2005;3:154–157.

10 Stern ME, Pflugfelder SC: Inflammation in dry eye. Ocul Surf 2004;2:124–130.

11 Gilbard JP, Farris RL: Tear osmolarity and ocular surface disease in keratoconjunctivitis sicca. Arch Ophthalmol 1979;97:1642–1646.

12 Gilbard JP: Tear film osmolarity and keratoconjunctivitis sicca. CLAO J 1985;11:243–250.

13 Farris RL, Gilbard JP, Stuchell RN, Mandel ID: Diagnostic tests in keratoconjunctivitis sicca. CLAO J 1983;9:23–28.

14 Gilbard JP, Farris RL, Santamaria J: Osmolarity of tear microvolumes in keratoconjunctivitis sicca. Arch Ophthalmol 1978;96:677–681.

15 Gilbard JP: Human tear film electrolyte concentrations in health and dry-eye disease. Int Ophthalmol Clin 1994;34:27–36.

16 Tomlinson A, Khanal S, Ramaesh K, Diaper C, McFadyen A: Tear film osmolarity: determination of a referent for dry eye diagnosis. Invest Ophthalmol Vis Sci 2006;47:4309–4315.

17 Liu H, Begley C, Chen M, Bradley A, Bonanno J, McNamara NA, Nelson JD, Simpson T: A link between tear instability and hyperosmolarity in dry eye. Invest Ophthalmol Vis Sci 2009;50:3671–3679.

18 Mastman GJ, Baldes EJ, Henderson JW: The total osmotic pressure of tears in normal and various pathologic conditions. Arch Ophthalmol 1961;65:509–513.

19 Scherz W, Doane MG, Dohlman CH: Tear volume in normal eyes and keratoconjunctivitis sicca. Albrecht Von Graefes Arch Klin Exp Ophthalmol 1974;192:141–150.

PD Dr. Elisabeth M. Messmer
Department of Ophthalmology, Ludwig Maximilian University
Mathildenstrasse 8
DE–80336 Munich (Germany)
Tel. +49 89 5160 3811, Fax +49 89 5160 5160, E-Mail emessmer@med.uni-muenchen.de

Brewitt H (ed): Research Projects in Dry Eye Syndrome.
Dev Ophthalmol. Basel, Karger, 2010, vol 45, pp 139–147

Novel Ocular Lubricant Containing an Intelligent Delivery System: Details of Its Mechanism of Action

Clark Springs

Department of Ophthalmology, Indiana University, Indianapolis, Ind., USA

Abstract

Objective: The purpose of this review is to outline the mechanism of action of a novel ocular lubricant incorporating hydroxypropyl-guar (HPG) and the demulcents polyethylene glycol 400 and propylene glycol. **Methods:** The literature relating to the mechanism of action of Systane Ultra is presented. The literature search covered the period prior to June 2008. A manual search was also conducted based on citations in the published literature. Additional original reports were referenced if relevant to the subject matter of the review. **Results and Conclusion:** The published literature supports the efficacy of an ocular lubricant containing HPG at reducing the signs and symptoms of dry eye through its multiphasic behavior and duration of action. This new formulation presents an additional benefit of a delivery system to further reduce the assimilation time of the product on-eye. Beneficial outcomes have been documented for tear film interaction, blur profile, viscoelasticity and tensile strength.

Dry eye disease is a complex, multifactorial and highly prevalent ocular condition. Recent data indicate that approximately 20–30 million Americans suffer from dry eye [1]. Based on current living conditions and lifestyles as well as an aging population, dry eye disease is anticipated to significantly increase. It is estimated that over USD 1 billion per year is spent worldwide on treating dry eye conditions.

Studying dry eye disease and the design of effective treatments have proven difficult due to the multifactorial nature of the disease. Insight into dry eye disease classification and management has recently been addressed in a recent publication from the International Dry Eye Workshop [2]. As research continues in this area, day-to-day treatment of dry eye is often challenging for the practicing eye care professional (ECP). An understanding of the mechanism of action and proposed benefits of the over-the-counter and prescription products used for dry eye is essential for the ECP. Presented in this paper is a detailed description of the mechanism of action of a new artificial tear product.

Physiology of the Tear Film

The classical picture of the tear film is described as a trilaminar structure consisting of: (1) a mucin layer overlying the corneal epithelium; (2) an aqueous layer composed of proteins and proteoglycans including soluble mucins; (3) a lipid layer at the tear-air interface [3]. Current opinion suggests that the structure of the tear film is complex and the layers are not discrete, but rather have interactive functionality. For example, the aqueous layer is now recognized to contain, in addition to ions, a variety of polyelectrolyte proteins which can interact with the superficial lipid layer to generate interfacial molecular structures that impart stability to the tear film [4–6]. In addition, Mugdil et al. [7] found the protein lysozyme usually present in the aqueous, to also be present at the surface of the tear film where it contributes to decreasing the surface tension through adsorption and penetration of meibomian lipids for further stability of the tear film.

Tear mucins are glycoproteins with high molecular weights ranging from 0.5 to 20 MDa. Normal tears contain predominantly membrane-bound and secretory mucins. They also contain soluble (monomeric) mucins. The membrane-bound (or transmembrane) mucins have increased residence time at boundaries of the cells generating them, the ocular epithelial cells. These mucins are intrinsic to the glycocalyx, interacting with the tear film to enhance wettability as well as providing a barrier to abrasion and invasion. Secretory and gel-forming mucins, produced by goblet cells, provide shear-dependent viscoelasticity for reduced viscosity during a blink and increased viscosity between blinks for greater tear film stability. The lacrimal and accessory lacrimal glands generate primarily soluble mucins along with the major volume of the tears. The properties of mucin are often emulated in over-the-counter artificial tear solutions with the inclusion of polymers possessing shear-dependent characteristics.

Dry Eye Management

Artificial tears are the most commonly used treatment for the signs and symptoms of dry eye [8]. These aqueous solutions of different formulations comprising soluble polymers are designed to improve lubrication of the ocular surface and increase tear film stability [9, 10]. These polymers include cellulose derivatives such as hydroxypropyl methylcellulose, carboxymethylcellulose, HPG and hyaluronic acid. Oil-water emulsion products are also available (table 1). Early formulations of artificial tears, based primarily on cellulose derivatives, tend to have a transient effect on tear film stability [3] due to a relatively brief period of ocular retention. More viscous solutions increase residence time [11], yet have a tendency to blur vision upon instillation [12]. The introduction of HPG as a gelling agent in artificial tears has allowed formulations to exhibit viscoelastic and tribological (evaluation of friction) properties. These

Table 1. Commonly used artificial tear preparations

	Key component	Preservative	Usage	Manufacturer
Refresh Tears®	CMC	purite	1–2 drops as needed	Allergan
Tears Naturale®	HPMC	Polyquad	1–2 drops as needed	Alcon
GenTeal®	HPMC	sodium perborate	1–2 drops as needed	Novartis
Bion® Tears	HPMC and dextran 70	none	as often as needed	Alcon
Optive™	Glycerin and CMC	purite	1–2 drops as needed	Allergan
Systane®	PEG 400 and PG with HPG	Polyquad	1–2 drops as needed	Alcon
Blink Tears™	hyaluronic acid	OcuPure™		AMO

CMC = Carboxymethylcellulose; HPMC = hydroxypropyl methylcellulose; PEG 400 = polyethylene glycol 400; PG = propylene glycol.

properties can be optimized to allow for increased ocular retention time of the active ingredients while maintaining minimal blur upon instillation [13, 14].

HPG: Properties and Characteristics

In its natural form, guar is a plant-derived polysaccharide gum with a linear backbone of mannose units and side chains of galactose [15]. Because of its tendency to form a viscous gel through inter-chain hydrogen bonding, guar has a history of use as an excipient and a thickening agent in the food and pharmaceutical industries. Guar treated with alkaline propylene oxide yields HPG, which is readily hydrated and easier to dissolve [16–19] than native guar. HPG is favored in many industrial applications to prolong the efficacy of active ingredients [15]. HPG is pH-sensitive due to the condensation reaction of borate onto the guar backbone. Borate ion concentrations increase with pH and the availability of borate at pH >7 will lead to cross-linking and subsequent gelation of the polymer. Factors that control the gelation process include the HPG and borate concentrations and the pH.

Use of HPG in the Treatment of Dry Eye

The gelling properties of HPG are well suited for use in artificial tear preparations and have advanced the treatment options for the ECP. Systane® Lubricant Eye Drops (Alcon

Laboratories, Fort Worth, Texas, USA) contain the demulcents polyethylene glycol 400 (PEG 400) and propylene glycol (PG), the gelling agent HPG, the buffer borate and the preservative Polyquad 0.001%. HPG interacts with borate ions in solution differently depending on the pH. At a pH of 7.0, the pH of the solution in the bottle, the solution exhibits low viscosity. However, once exposed to the pH of the ocular tears (pH of approximately 7.5) [20], the HPG cross-links with borate and increases in viscosity to form a thin gel with bio-adhesive properties for retention of the demulcents on the ocular surface [19, 21]. It appears that the large HPG molecules preferentially associate at more hydrophobic zones in the tear film (i.e. at compromised areas of epithelium where the glycocalyx is no longer intact) [22], thereby providing a protective coating over the ocular surface that facilitates healing and lubricates the eye [19, 23].

Clinical Efficacy of an HPG-Containing Ocular Lubricant

Ubels et al. [19] showed that artificial tears containing HPG facilitate corneal epithelial cell recovery in vivo and provide long-term desiccation protection of the intact cornea both in vivo and in vitro. To investigate the effect of different eye drops on reducing the coefficient of friction, Meyer et al. [24] tested various eye drops on stabilized umbilical vein tissue. Systane showed a significant reduction in the coefficient of friction compared to the other artificial tears tested ($p < 0.01$).

In clinical studies, it has been shown that Systane produces a significant ($p < 0.0001$ at day 28) improvement in the signs and symptoms of moderate dry eye disease [25]. Results from Gifford et al. [12] concur with a reduction in symptoms of ocular discomfort and in ocular staining scores in dry eye patients after 4 weeks. Christensen et al. [22] found Systane to have even greater efficacy in patients with higher levels of baseline corneal staining, indicating a contribution to corneal recovery. Moreover, the authors suggest that regular use of Systane promotes natural tissue repair. Cervan-Lopez et al. [26] found that use of Systane facilitated epithelial regeneration and thus enhanced barrier function.

Christensen et al. [22], in a 6-week study, found that Systane showed statistically significant improvements in the signs (corneal and conjunctival staining) and symptoms of dry eye ($p = 0.015$ in the morning and $p = 0.023$ in the evening) compared to another commercially available lubricating solution containing carboxymethylcellulose. With Systane, both corneal and conjunctival staining were significantly reduced ($p = 0.024$ and $p = 0.025$ respectively), with a 52% reduction in corneal staining compared to baseline and a statistically significant treatment effect shown for conjunctival staining compared to the carboxymethylcellulose-containing solution ($p = 0.025$).

Systane has demonstrated a significant effect on extension of the tear film break-up time with significant increases after instillation of the drop reported by Christensen et al. [27], Pollard et al. [28] (in a pilot study), Guillon et al. [29] and Gifford et al. [12]. Systane also showed statistically significant extensions in tear film break-up time compared to lubricating solutions containing carboxymethylcellulose and glycerin/polysorbate, presumably due to the HPG borate complex [27, 29–31].

A key requirement of artificial tears, besides lubrication and tear film stability, is that they have minimal effect on vision immediately after instillation. While this has been an issue for most artificial tears to some degree, those that have greater viscosity tend to exhibit greater blurring. Systane, with its ability to remain a liquid on initial contact with the eye and to subsequently form a gel on-eye serves to minimize blur on contact while providing greater viscosity in situ [22]. Based on the finding that transient blurred vision is the main adverse event reported with PEG/PG lubricant eye drops, it has been proposed that certain individuals may have a predisposition to blur based on the pH of their natural tears. While the average tear pH is approximately 7.5, the range of normal ocular pH values lies between 7.1 and 7.8. This may account for the infrequent/inconsistent reports of subjective blur immediately after instillation with Systane [12].

New Formulation Systane Ultra

Systane® Ultra Lubricant Eye Drops (Alcon Laboratories) contain PEG 400 and PG as demulcents in solution with HPG as the gelling agent. Borate and sorbitol are key ingredients in the formulation. The multidose preparation is preserved with Polyquad [32]. Sorbitol is a water-soluble non-ionic compound often used as a tonicity adjustment agent. Sorbitol, in Systane Ultra, competes with the HPG in complexing with borate [16] in order to control viscosity in the bottle for effective delivery in the eye. The addition of sorbitol allows for efficient spreading upon instillation to the eye. The mechanism of action of the technology, from the bottle to contact with the eye and tear film mixing, is described below.

Mechanism of Action of Systane Ultra

In the bottle, at a pH of 7.9, the weakly cross-linked sorbitol-borate-HPG complexes are in a state of dynamic equilibrium. In applying the weakly structured gel to the eye, the pressure exerted on the bottle to extract a drop creates a reduction in the gel viscosity due to 'shear thinning'. Ketelson et al. [13] demonstrated that the relationship between the shear stress and the strain rate are nonlinear (non-newtonian) with Systane Ultra. The non-newtonian property is designated since the flow properties cannot be described by a single constant value of viscosity. As this relates to the delivery to the ocular surface, the high shear rate exhibited by Systane Ultra allows for very low viscosity upon instillation and immediately after blinks. The resultant drop delivered to the eye is a liquid with non-newtonian characteristics. It is during this time that the conditions of the ocular environment influence the chemistry of the solution. In the tear film, the low-molecular-weight hydrophilic sorbitol dissociates from the borate and is diluted in the tear film, minimizing the critical effect it exerted in the bottle in controlling viscosity. The HPG is then able to complex with free borate ions, increasing the cross-link density and subsequently the liquid viscosity to form a gel

[15]. Other factors in the ocular environment that also play a role in enhancing the cross-linked network and adhesion properties in the eye include the pH 7.5 (SD ± 0.23) [20], and the presence of natural divalent ions in the tear film [15]. The change in tonicity as the solution mixes with the tears as well as the interaction of tear-based divalent ions increase the strength of the cross-linked network and retention in the eye. The presence of calcium ions in the tear film in particular appears to have a key role in increasing the strength of the network [33]. The interaction of the solution with the tear film creates a matrix on the ocular surface allowing the retention of HPG and the demulcents.

Recent Clinical Findings

Laboratory testing by Lu et al. [15], analyzing the association of HPG and borate to the tear film, has shown that the HPG-borate complexes behave as negatively-charged macromolecules (polyelectrolytes) that slowly complex with cationic lysozyme at pH 7.8. These molecular interactions verify that pH and electrostatic attraction contribute to the close association of the HPG-borate complex with the tear film constituents for retention of the introduced components on the eye.

Systane Ultra is expected to demonstrate the same behavioral characteristics attributable to the HPG on-eye as in original Systane with respect to lubricity, affinity for the epithelium, retention on the ocular surface, ocular surface protection and restoration of ocular health [19, 21, 22, 27, 34–37].

Meadows et al. [38] evaluated changes in solution characteristics relating to lubricity of Systane Ultra. Under conditions simulating initial introduction to the eye, the formulation was found to decrease in viscosity and in elastic modulus with a reduction in pH from 7.9 to 7.6. A subsequent increase in viscoelasticity and a significant reduction in friction occurred when the formulation was modified to simulate dilution in the eye. Experiments on rheology (defined as the study of the flow of matter) at the tear film interface showed lysozyme and mucin had an additional synergistic effect on increasing the elastic moduli of this novel lubricating eye drop for long-lasting lubrication and surface protection in the eye.

Ketelson et al. [13] measured the extensional rheology properties of HPG solutions to model the properties of Systane Ultra when dropped into the eye. The data showed significant extension in long filament break-up times in a simulated dilution experiment. Extensional viscosities decreased slightly after decreasing the pH from 7.9 to 7.6 and then extensional elasticity dramatically increased after dilution of the sorbitol, indicating increased tensile strength. The extensional rheological properties of Systane Ultra appear to be an important physical property that may benefit and improve tear film stability.

A two-period crossover, single-dose per period study involving 20 dry eye patients comparing Systane Ultra to Optive® (Allergan, Inc., Irvine, Calif., USA) investigated the blur profile immediately after instillation of the 2 ocular lubricants (fig. 1). Initially, and through the first 90 s after instillation, there was no clinically significant

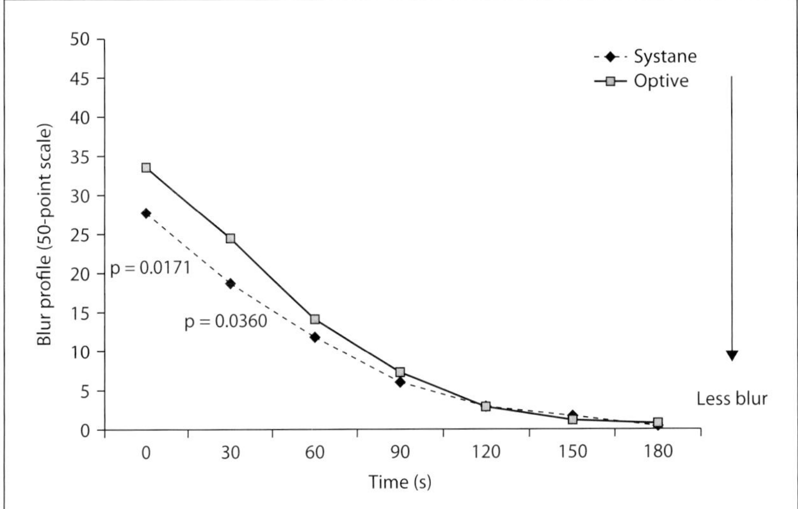

Fig. 1. Blur profile.

difference in blur between Systane Ultra and Optive, supporting the notion that Systane maintains reduced viscosity when it is required and that the subsequent gelation is controlled [14].

Conclusion

The published literature supports the efficacy of an ocular lubricant containing HPG at reducing the signs and symptoms of dry eye through its multiphasic behavior and duration of action. A new formulation, Systane Ultra, presents an additional benefit of a delivery system to further reduce the assimilation time of the product on the eye. It exhibits non-newtonian characteristics, with low shear and viscosity upon instillation. Once on the eye, the elastic modulus and viscoelastic properties allow for retention of the active ingredients and a low coefficient of friction during the blink process. Superior outcomes have been documented for tear film interaction, blur profile, viscoelasticity and tensile strength, suggesting a beneficial lubricant eye drop product for dry eye patients.

Acknowledgment

The author thanks Lauren Richard, B.Optom, for her medical writing contributions.

References

1 Moss SE, Klein R, Klein BE: Prevalence of and risk factors for dry eye syndrome. Arch Ophthalmol 2000;118:1264–1268.

2 The definition and classification of dry eye disease: report of the Definition and Classification Subcommittee of the International Dry Eye WorkShop. Ocul Surf 2007;5:75–92.

3 Holly FJ: Wettability and bioadhesion in Ophthalmology; in Schrader ME, Loeb GI (eds): Modern Approaches to Wettability. New York, Plenum Press, 1992.

4 Gasymov OK, Abduragimov AR, Yusifov TN, Glasgow BJ: Binding studies of tear lipocalin: the role of conserved tryptophan in maintaining structure, stability and ligand affinity. Biochim Biophys Acta 1999;1433:307–320.

5 Glasgow BJ, Marshall G, Gasymov OK, Abduragimov AR, Yusifov TN, Knobler CM: Tear lipocalins: potential lipid scavengers for the corneal surface. Invest Ophthalmol Vis Sci 1999;40:3100–3107.

6 Nagyova B, Tiffany JM: Components responsible for the surface tension of human tears. Curr Eye Res 1999;19:4–11.

7 Mugdil P, Torres M, Millar T: Adsoption of lysozyme to phospholipid and meibomian lipid monolayer films. Colloids Surf B Biointerfaces 2006;48:128–137.

8 Aragona P, Papa V, Micali A, Santocono M, Milazzo G: Long term treatment with sodium hyaluronate-containing artificial tears reduces ocular surface damage in patients with dry eye. Br J Ophthalmol 2002;86:181–184.

9 Oechsner M, Keipert S: Polyacrylic acid/polyvinylpyrrolidone bipolymeric systems. I. Rheological and mucoadhesive properties of formulations potentially useful for the treatment of dry-eye-syndrome. Eur J Pharm Biopharm 1999;47:113–118.

10 Smart JD, Kellaway IW, Worthington HE: An in-vitro investigation of mucosa-adhesive materials for use in controlled drug delivery. J Pharm Pharmacol 1984;36:295–299.

11 Gilbard JP: Nutrition and the eye: dry eye and the role of nutrition. Optom Today 2004;June:34–39.

12 Gifford P, Evans BJW, Morris J: A clinical evaluation of Systane. Contact Lens Ant Eye 2006;29:31–40.

13 Ketelson HA, Davis J, Meadows DL: Extensional rheological properties of an artificial tear delivery system. Poster, ARVO, 2008.

14 Christensen MT, Martin AE, David RE: A comparison of comfort/acceptability and blur profile between PEG/PG and CMC/glycerin based artificial tears in both a dry eye and non-dry eye patient populations. Poster, ARVO, 2008.

15 Lu C, Kostanski L, Ketelson H, Meadows D, Pelton R: Hydroxypropyl guar-borate interactions with tear film mucin and lysozyme. Langmuir 2005;21: 10032–10037.

16 Kasvan S, Prud'homme RK: Rheology of guar and HP-guar crosslinked by borate. Macromolecules 1992;25:2026–2032.

17 Pezon E, Ricard A, Lafuma F, Audebert R: Reversible gel formation induced by ion complexation. 1. Borax–galactomannan interaction. Macromolecules 1988;21:1121–1125.

18 Cheng Y, Brown KM, Prud'homme RK: Characterization and intermolecular interactions of hydroxypropyl guar solutions. Biomacromolecules 2002;3:456–461.

19 Ubels JL, Clousing DP, Van Haitsma TA, Hong BS, Stauffer P, Asgharian B, Meadows D: Pre clinical investigation of the efficacy of an artificial tear solution containing hydroxypropyl-guar as a gelling agent. Curr Eye Res 2004;28:437–444.

20 Yamada M, Mochizuki H, Kawai M, Yoshino M, Mashima Y: Fluorophotometric measurement of pH of human tears in vivo. Curr Eye Res 1997;16: 482–486.

21 Khurana AK, Chaaudhary R, Ahluwalia BK, Gupta S: Tear film profile in dry eye. Acta Ophthalmologica 1991;9:79–86.

22 Christensen MT, Cohen S, Rinehart J, Akers F, Pemberton B, Bloomenstein M, Lesher M, Kaplan D, Meadows D, Meuse P, Hearn C, Stein JM: Clinical evaluation of an HP-guar gellable lubricant eye drop for the relief of dryness of the eye. Curr Eye Res 2004;28:55–62.

23 Korb DR, Herman JP, Greiner JV, Scaffidi RC, Finnemore VM, Exford JM, Blackie CA, Douglass T: Lid wiper epitheliopathy and dry eye symptoms. Eye Contact Lens 2005;31:2–8.

24 Meyer AE, Baier RE, Chen H, Chowham M: Differential tissue-on-tissue lubrication by ophthalmic formulations. J Biomed Mater Res B Appl Biomater 2007;82:74–88.

25 Hartstein I, Khwarg S, Przydryga J: An open-label evaluation of HP-Guar gellable lubricant eye drops for the improvement of dry eye signs and symptoms in a moderate dry eye adult population. Curr Med Res Opin 2005;21:255–260.

26 Cervan-Lopez I, Saenz-Frances-San-Baldomero F, Benitez-Del-Castillo JM: Reduction of corneal permeability in patients treated with HP-Guar: a fluorometric study. Arch Soc Esp Oftalmol 2006;81: 327–332.

27 Christensen MT, Stein JM, Stone RP, Meadows DL: Evaluation of the effect on tear film break-up time extension by artificial tears in dry eye patients. Presentation, 23rd Biennial Cornea Res Conf, Boston, October 3–4, 2003.
28 Pollard S, Stone RP, Christensen MT, Ousler GW, Abelson MB: Extension in tear film break-up time after instilation of HP-guar artificial tear substitute. Invest Ophthalmol Vis Sci 2003;44:E-abstract 2489.
29 Guillon M, Chamberlain P, Marks MG, Stein JM: Effect of eye drop compositional characteristics on tear film. Paper, ARVO Ann Meet, Fort Lauderdale, April 28, 2004.
30 Carels I, Stone RP, Stein JM, Christensen MT, Meadows DL, Przydryga J: Prolonged tear film break up time using a new ocular lubricating drop that gels in the eye. Poster, EVER, 2003.
31 Ousler GW, Michaelson C, Christensen MT: An evaluation of tear film breakup time extension and ocular protection index scores among three marketed lubricant eye drops. Cornea 2007;26:949–952.
32 Tripathi BJ, Tripathi RC, Kolli SP: Cytotoxicity of ophthalmic preservatives on human corneal epithelium. Lens Eye Toxic Res 1992;9:361–375.
33 Hägerström H, Paulsson M, Edsman K: Evaluation of mucoadhesion for two polyelectrolyte gels in simulated physiological conditions using a rheological method. Eur J Pharm Sci 2000;9:301–309.
34 Ketelson H, Meadows DL, McQueen N, Stone R: The effect of black copolymer surfactants and tear components on the dynamic wettability properties of contact lenses and tear film stability. Paper, Colloids and Surfaces: Biointerfaces, Baltimore, October 27, 2004.
35 Hong B, Stauffer P, Meadows DL, Stone R: Desiccation protection capability of various demulcents in artificial tear formulations. Paper, ARVO Ann Meet, Fort Lauderdale, May 6, 2003.
36 Asgharian B, Nolen L, Meadows DL, Stone R: Novel gel-forming ophthalmic polymer system for artificial tear solution. Paper, ARVO Ann Meet, Fort Lauderdale, May 6, 2003.
37 Meadows DL, Ubels JL, Aupperlee MD: Efficacy of artificial tears for protection of the corneal epithelium from desiccation. Paper, ARVO Ann Meet, Fort Lauderdale, May 8, 2002.
38 Meadows DL, Ketelson HA, Davis J: Characterization of a novel polymeric artificial tear delivery system. Poster, ARVO, 2008.

Clark Springs, MD
Department of Ophthalmology, Indiana University
200 W. 103rd Street No. 2200
Indianapolis, IN 46290 (USA)
Tel. +1 317 278 5100, Fax +1 317 278 5101, E-Mail csprings@iupui.edu

Author Index

Subject Index

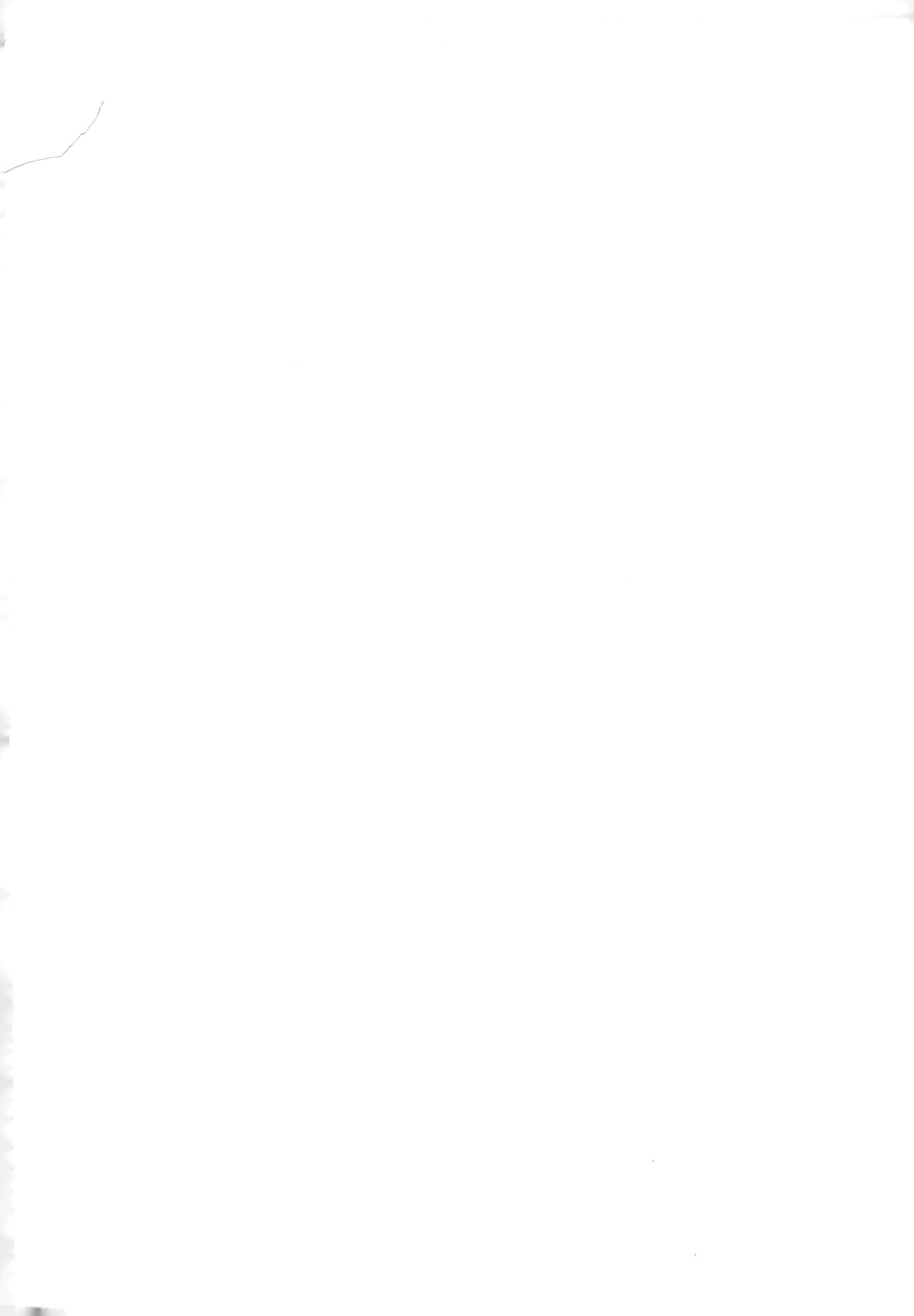